Praise for *Penis Power*

"Finally, an easy and practical approach to male sexuality. *Penis Power* is the book that every man (and woman) will go to when questions arise about the performer and the act of the performance."

> —David Y. Josephson, MD, Program Director, Urologic Oncology and Robotic Surgery Fellowship, City of Hope National Medical Center

"Dr. Danoff, a world-class urologist, has written a world-class book that should be read by every man and woman who enjoys sex."

> —Wolfgang Puck, restaurateur and world-famous chef, Spago

"A great book. *Penis Power* is a must-read for all men and women who love sex!"

> —Mancow Muller, host, *Mancow Experience*, WABC Talk Radio

"Dr. Danoff brings forward his deep knowledge and experience as a leading urologist in an educational and entertaining book that should address every question that most men utter only inside the confines of their doctors' exam rooms. I should tell you that their wives and girlfriends ask me the same questions, and this book is a great resource for them as well."

> —Sharron L. Mee, MD, Female Urologist

"A must-read for all men who care about their physical and sexual health."

> —Joe Weider, world-famous bodybuilder, fitness guru, and publisher of *Men's Fitness*

"A stimulating and educational medical guide that will renew men's lives in the bedroom and keep them out of the operating room."

> —Stuart Holden, MD, Medical Director, Prostate Cancer Foundation

"Insightful, educational, and liberating—this book is going to help a lot of people."

—Bill Paxton

"Simply the most empowering book of the millennium—a mastery of storytelling."

—Christopher S. Ng, MD, Chief, Division of Urology, Cedars-Sinai Medical Center

"At last it is great to see a volume that produces such a constant flow of information. The information fills nearly every void on the subject and finally exposes the long and short of it."

—Johnny Mathis

"One of the best books I have ever read on male sexual health; extremely well written, easy to understand, informative, and lighthearted."

—George DeJohn, host, *Train Station Fitness Show*, SportsRadio, and creator, 21 Day Body Makeover

"Where was this book when I was growing up? I could have been Superman instead of Caspar Milquetoast!"

—Terence Kingsley-Smith, writer

"*Penis Power* is definitely original. It's also clever, informative, and entertaining."

—Ron Clark, playwright

"A book loaded with wisdom and wit, masterfully written by Dr. Dudley Seth Danoff. I recommend this book highly as a happy Dr. Danoff patient. For over thirty-five years, he has kept my 'below the belt' confidence high and my PSA low."

—Jerry Mayer, playwright and television writer and producer

Penis Power

The Ultimate Guide to Male Sexual Health

Also by the author

Superpotency: How to Get It, Use It, and Maintain It for a Lifetime

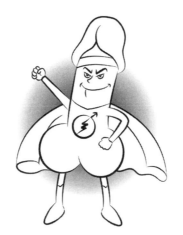

Penis Power

The Ultimate Guide to Male Sexual Health

Dudley Seth Danoff, MD, FACS

DEL MONACO PRESS

Beverly Hills, California

Del Monaco Press
369 S. Doheny Drive, #113
Beverly Hills, CA 90211
www.delmonacopress.com

Ordering Information

Orders by U.S. trade bookstores and wholesalers. Please contact Independent Publishers Group, 814 North Franklin Street, Chicago, IL 60610. Tel: (312) 337-0747; Fax (312) 337-5985, www.ipgbook.com.Printed in the United States of America

Cataloging-in-Publication data

Danoff, Dudley Seth.
    Penis power : the ultimate guide to male sexual health / Dudley Seth Danoff, MD.
    p. cm.
    Includes index.
    ISBN 978-0-9831998-3-0
    1. Sexual health. 2. Penis. 3. Sexual health. 4. Men --Sexual behavior. 5. Penis --Physiology. 6. Erectile dysfunction. 7. Prostate --Diseases --Popular works. I. Title.
    HQ56 .D21 2011
    613.9/6 --dc22   2011928210

First Edition

15 14 13 12 11   10 9 8 7 6 5 4 3 2 1

Medical Disclaimer

The information contained in this book is intended for educational purposes only and is not intended for the treatment or prevention of disease or as a substitute for medical treatment or as an alternative to medical advice. Should you have any healthcare related questions or concerns please contact your physician or other qualified healthcare provider promptly.

Every attempt has been made to present accurate and timely information. The author and publisher assume neither liability nor responsibility to any person or entity with respect to any direct or indirect loss or damage caused, or alleged to be caused, by the information contained herein, or for errors, omissions, inaccuracies, or any other inconsistency within these pages, or for unintentional slights against people or organizations. The author and publisher are not associated with any manufacturers of the products mentioned and are not guaranteeing the safety of these products.

While the publisher and author have used their best efforts in preparing this book, they make no representations or warranties with respect to the accuracy or completeness of the contents of this book and specifically disclaim any implied warranties for a particular purpose. The advice and strategies contained herein may not be suitable for your situation. You should consult with a professional where appropriate. Neither the publisher nor the author shall be liable for any loss of profit or any other commercial damages, including but not limited to special, incidental, consequential, or other damages. The information in this reference is not intended to substitute for expert medical advice or treatment. It is designed to help you make informed choices. Because each individual is unique, a physician or other qualified healthcare provider must diagnose conditions and supervise treatments for each individual health problem. If an individual is under the care of a doctor or other qualified healthcare practitioner or provider and receives advice contrary to information provided in this reference, the doctor or other qualified healthcare practitioner's advice should be followed, as it is based on the unique characteristics of that individual.

To my father—a man of true penis power

Contents

Preface   xi

Part 1 Everything You Need to Know about the Penis

Chapter 1: Maximizing Your Penis Power   3
  Men Are Penis-Oriented Creatures   4
  We Are Tragically Ill-Informed about the Penis   7
  An Epidemic of Penis Weakness   10
  Why Are We Having This Epidemic Now?   14
  A Wake-Up Call   21
  The Secret of Penis Power   22

Chapter 2: The Truth about Penis Size   25
  Looks Are Not Everything   26
  One Size Fits All   28
  Your Penis Is Not Too Small   30
  Penis Power Is Not Related to Penis Size   31
  You Are as Big as You Think You Are   35
  The Big Myth: Penile Enhancement, Phalloplasty,
    and Penile Enlargement   37

Chapter 3: Erection and Ejaculation   41
  Erections: Whatever Turns You On   42
  Tumescence: Stand Up and Be Counted   45
  Orgasms: Come Again?   46
  Semen: From Whence It Comes   47
  The Point of No Return   49
  The Refractory Period: I Want to Be Alone   51

Chapter 4: Medical Conditions That Affect Penis Power   55
  Impotence: "My Friend Has This Problem . . ."   56
  The Nerve of It: Neurological Disorders   62
  When It Cannot Go with the Flow: Vascular Disorders   63
  A Little Prick for a Big Reward: Injectable Drugs   64

When Things Are Not Quite Right: Hormonal Disorders   65
Steroids: Big Biceps and Tiny Testes   67
Do Not Be Sicker Than You Really Are   68
Prescription Medications: Is the Pharmacist Really Your
    Enemy?   70
It's Not All Fun and Games: Recreational Drugs   73
Premature Ejaculation   75

Chapter 5: Prostatic and Other Urologic Diseases   83
BPH: Don't Panic!   83
Alternatives to a Prostatectomy   86
Prostate Cancer   90
Testicular Cancer: The Lance Armstrong Theory   95
Kidney Transplants   96
The Good News   97

Chapter 6: Blue Pills and Other Medical Cures for Erectile
    Dysfunction   99
Blue Magic: The Saga of "the Pills" for Men   99
It's Not Candy   101
Use with Caution   102
You Are Not Alone   104
Do Not Let the Hype Fool You   106
From Pills to Pellets: The Muse System   107
Shooting It Up: Injectable Medication   109
Surgical Procedures   113
Pump It Up: Implants   114
Mechanical Devices   118
Aphrodisiacs and Other Substances   119

Chapter 7: Performance Anxiety: When It's All in Your Head   123
Anxiety Is Penis Power's Archenemy   126
Accentuate the Positive   126
Even the Strong Are Let Down Sometimes   128
Lighten Up, Dude   131
Don't Worry, Be Superpotent   135
Depression Depresses the Penis   139

Mind Games 140
Fears 142

Chapter 8: Extenuating Circumstances: When Sex
Becomes a Chore 145
The Hard Dick Syndrome 147
The Spice of Life 150
Hard on Demand 152
Be Careful! 153
"Blow" Is Not an Accurate Description 154
A Time and Place for Everything 156
The Sweet Smell of Success 158
The Most Unpleasant Aspect of Sex 160
Intimate Intimidation 162
When the Problem Is in Your Heart 165

Chapter 9: As Old as You Feel: The Life Story of the Penis 169
Penis Passages 171
The Early Years 173
Is It Ageless? 174
When the Going Gets Tough: Male Menopause and TRT 178
Who Needs Testosterone Replacement? 179
Good News, but at a Price 180
Young at Heart, Young in Person 183
Andropause versus Menopause 185
Penis Posterity 186
Sex in the New Millennium 188

Chapter 10: Sexually Transmitted Diseases 189
Chlamydia: Silent but Troublesome 190
Gonorrhea: This Clap Is Not a Cheer 191
Syphilis: Next to AIDS, the Worst of All 191
Genital Herpes: Not the Scourge of the Twenty-First
Century 192
AIDS: *The* Scourge of the Twenty-First Century 193

Chapter 11: What Women Need to Know 197
Ladies and Gentlemen: It Begins with Communication 199

Women's Top Ten Complaints   201

Penis-Oriented Women Have More Fun   209

Chapter 12: Penis FAQs   211

Part 2 Becoming a Superpotent Man

Chapter 13: What's Your Penis Personality?   237

Positive Penis Personalities   240

Negative Penis Personalities   249

Chapter 14: What Is a Superpotent Man?   265

Discovering Penis Power   266

The Character of the Superpotent Man   268

The Superpotent Man and Sex   273

Penis Power Is Defined by Who You Are and How

You Control Your Life   284

Chapter 15: How to Become a Superpotent Man   287

Educate Yourself   288

Good Health Equals Good Penis Power   290

Penis Power Exercises   294

Maybe Elvis Was on to Something: Pelvic Control   295

The Harder They Come: Controlling Your Timing   296

The "Tain't" Exercises   300

Techniques for Delaying Ejaculation   301

Eliminate Negativity and Self-Doubt   304

Do Not View Sex as a Performance   306

Make Friends with Your Penis   307

A Final Word to Women   308

A Final Word to Men   308

Acknowledgments   311

Notes   313

Index   317

About the Author   329

Preface

I have been a practicing urologist for more than thirty years. It was a little more than ten years ago when I first made the disturbing observation that an increasing number of American men were suffering from what I call "penis weakness."

At that time, there was very little discussion within the urologic community about the significance of this problem in male genital health. As I looked deeper into the issue, it struck me that as much as the stigma of penis weakness was plaguing men in modern times, it had probably been plaguing men throughout all of history.

I began to speak out and write about the principal characteristics of this pandemic. In so doing, I discovered a deeper reality about men and their relationships to their penises. I learned that the vast majority of males have suffered from some form of penis weakness: physical, psychological, or both.

The most significant aspect of the penis weakness phenomenon is that its debilitating effects are, in most cases, compounded by a lack of knowledge by both men and women. For too many years, men who have suffered from the self-doubt and anxiety caused by penis weakness have done so without any guidance from the medical community in general and shockingly little significant support from the professional urologic community in particular.

I realized something had to be done. What resulted was the book *Superpotency*—an all-inclusive guide to overcoming the medical and psychological factors that lead to penis weakness.

That book was supposed to be titled *Penis Power*. The year was 1993. I thought those two words would be a revolutionary title for a book on male sexual health. What I discovered, however, was that, according to my editors, it was a little *too* revolutionary. The book was not published under that title because the publisher (Warner Books) felt that no legitimate, mainstream book on male genital health by a credible author could have the controversial word *penis* in the title. With a nod to political correctness, the publisher and I settled for the less explosive title *Superpotency*. This was prior to Howard Stern, the Lorena Bobbitt affair, the Pamela Anderson and Tommy Lee videos, the plays *Vagina Monologues* and *Puppetry of the Penis*, satellite radio, the Internet, and Viagra, Cialis, and Levitra commercials in every sports facility in the country. Now, how can I shy away from a title that includes the word *penis* when every five minutes we are warned: "If your erection lasts longer than four hours, call your doctor!"?

Oh, how things have changed.

Or have they?

After much deliberation, the book *Superpotency* finally hit book-shelves in the United States and around the world. Ultimately, it would come to be printed in more than twelve languages. Thousands of copies were sold to men *and* women, straight couples, gay couples, and everyone in between. The overwhelming response from the public was that the vital information contained in the book generated a sense of sexual enlightenment. Those individuals and couples who shared the knowledge of the book developed the skills and the confidence to address the problematic issues surrounding male genital health and sexual potency. The important information about male sexual health I set out to share had become the cornerstone for a new phase of the sexual revolution.

Fast-forward to 2011.

Penis weakness is still rampant throughout the world. With the advent of major pharmaceutical drugs designed to aid erectile dys-

function and their international advertising campaigns, some of
the significant issues in male genital health have suddenly become
part of the general social consciousness. It is still astonishing that,
in my medical practice, insecurity and uncertainty about sexual
performance are the top problems for my patients. Most of them
are totally uninformed about the nature of their penises and their
bodies in general. They are also frighteningly misinformed about
the medical resources available today.

As a physician and a husband, I am saddened to see how many
men and their partners deprive themselves of the complete sexual
satisfaction and enjoyment they deserve. Fortunately, over the
past decade, monumental advances in the treatment of erectile
dysfunction, prostate cancer, and other urologic conditions have
been made. There is a new openness in attitude toward the penis
in general. Indeed, the penis is *almost* out of the closet. With the
dawn of this new cultural and technological era, I saw the need to
recreate the original concept of the book: to replace ignorance and
mythology with factual information and to replace self-doubt with
confidence.

My goal, as it has always been, is to help every man realize,
achieve, and maximize his penis power.

I have seen more than two hundred thousand patient penises
in my professional lifetime. While each is unique, just as hands and
feet are unique, all are also remarkably alike anatomically. More important, there is enormous variation in *how* each functions in its
sexual capacity. I have observed that these differences in functional
ability and capacity have very little to do with the anatomy of a
particular penis or even with a man's physical size, looks, or level of
success, wealth, and status. Mainly, they have to do with how men
perceive their own penises. In addition to understanding its biological functions, every man must learn that the penis is an organ of
expression. What gives it its power is much more than the condition of its blood vessels and nerves.

Penis power is a transformative concept based on positive thinking.

Applying the power of positive thought to your penis can change your entire life.

Your penis is what you *think* it is.

- It is as *big* as you think it is.
- It is as *reliable* as you think it is.
- It is as *potent* as you think it is.

This is the message of *Penis Power*.

This book is based on my medical observations and experience as a urologic surgeon and clinician for more than thirty years. Its goal is to help you achieve your full sexual potential. Even though one of my objectives is to educate the public, this is not a textbook. There is nothing overly technical in these pages. Rather, I have tried to express myself in straightforward, easily understandable terms. I have covered the facts about the penis and its related organs that I consider essential for both men and women to know. The amount that even well-educated, sophisticated people do not know about the penis is astounding. Even more shocking is what they *think* is true but is not.

Penis Power is not a psychology textbook either. Plenty of writers have given us lengthy analyses on male sexuality and treatises on the treatment of sexual dysfunction. My purpose is less academic and more practical. I am concerned with average men, men who are misinformed or confused about their penises, and extraordinary men who think they know everything but still have a lot to learn. When it comes to the penis, all men are the same: just *men*. Ultimately, this book is concerned with the attitudes and beliefs of men as sexual beings and the direct relationship between their personal attitudes and their penis attitudes.

This is not a "how-to" book in the mechanical sense. *Penis Power* is not a sex manual, though you will find many practical tips within these pages. These tips include exercises and lifestyle changes for improving penis power, sexual control, and confidence and instructions on how to achieve a healthy and active sex life with mental and physical happiness.

I want all of my readers to become penis experts. You will learn all there is to know about the male genital system: how it works, how it does not work, why it does not work, and how to get it to work for you again and for as long as possible. The information contained in these pages will help you learn how to move away from viewing sex as a "performance" and move toward sex as an exciting and pleasurable experience. Anxiety over performance is the fastest route to penis weakness. Through these pages you will learn how to relax and enjoy the sensuality and gratification of being in control of intimate moments by never allowing yourself to become emotionally intimidated by the fear of being sexual with a partner.

Ultimately, I want every man to understand that no matter what his personal problems may be, as long as he is making the effort to learn how to fully express his sexual potential, he will overcome those physical and psychological barriers. He will become a superpotent man and he will develop *penis power*.

To gain control of your sexuality, you will learn to eliminate negativity and self-doubt. You will face your imperfections with honesty and a sense of humor. You will learn about penis power and the ways in which age can affect it. You will become aware that as long as you are able to breathe, move your extremities, maintain relative control over your bodily functions, sustain a positive outlook, and remain alert enough to identify the day of the week, you can continue to exercise your penis power indefinitely. You will learn that you do not stop having sex because you get old; you get old because you stop exercising your penis power.

The book contains a section on andropause, the male equivalent of menopause, and an important section on testosterone replacement therapy (TRT), including its benefits and risks. *Penis Power* will show you that the greatest aphrodisiac and ally of penis power is love itself. Its archenemy is anger, hostility, and hatred. You will also learn about medical treatments for urologic problems such as prostate cancer, testicular cancer, hormonal disorders, vascular disorders, and other biological conditions, including erectile dysfunction. I have also included a comprehensive section on common sexually transmitted diseases (STDs) with diagnoses and treatments, as well as essential, everyday information on HIV/AIDS.

Penis Power is a book I wish had been written a long time ago. It would have saved a lot of lives. It would have saved a lot of men from self-doubt and humiliation. It would have saved a lot of women from sexual frustration. It would have saved a lot of marriages and relationships.

As I wrote this book, I imagined myself speaking to both male and female readers, heterosexuals and homosexuals. Even though this is a book regarding male sexuality and male physiology, my fervent wish is that as many women read it as men. I have never met a woman who did not want to maximize the penis power of the man in her life. This book has the potential to give female readers an improved understanding of men in general, including their bodies and their sexuality. With this valuable information at their disposal, women will have the ability to achieve the utmost satisfaction from their partners. Chapter 11 addresses women specifically. To avoid repetition, I did not include important information covered earlier in the book. For this reason, I urge all women to read the *entire* book. *Penis Power* is designed for both sexes. I also want all of my readers to know that the information in this book is blind to individual sexual orientation. The principles presented can be enormously helpful to both heterosexual and homosexual relationships. The same principles apply to wives, husbands, girlfriends, boyfriends, or partners. I use these terms interchangeably when the discussion involves sexual activity.

As you read this book, don't be distracted by the pronouns I use to refer to men's partners. As a physician, I have treated men with female partners, men with male partners, and men with both. But as a writer I think it's awkward to keep writing "he or she" every time I refer to a man's partner. So when I'm not referring to a specific patient and his partner I have alternated pronouns: sometimes the partner in an example is male, sometimes female. As you read, think of your own partner and insert the appropriate pronoun. The advice in this book will improve your penis power with any partner.

A lot of information in these pages will surprise you. Some of it might shock or outrage you. I welcome whatever controversy might ensue. I firmly stand behind my observations with one purpose only: to end the plague of penis weakness and the attendant cynicism, despair, and frustration that prevent the sexual happiness that all men and women deserve. Harnessing penis power to achieve superpotency is not a luxury; it is the natural birthright of every man. Its full exercise will render our lives—male and female, young and old—more vigorous, healthier, and more enjoyable in every respect.

If you follow the advice in this book, you will find that every aspect of your life—work, play, and relationships—will be enriched. A simple shift in attitude and an adjustment in your behavior patterns can give you the strength and confidence you need to achieve happiness in your sex life and ultimately in every aspect of who you are as a human being.

Penis Power will instill in you the ability to achieve superpotency throughout your entire life. It will elevate the mind, the heart, and the spirit—not just the penis.

The man who has it is blessed, and so is the partner with whom he shares it.

Dudley Seth Danoff, MD, FACS

Part 1

Everything You Need to Know about the Penis

Chapter 1

Maximizing Your Penis Power

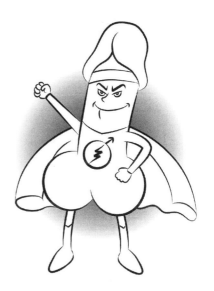

In the more than three decades that I have been practicing urology, I have treated every conceivable problem in the male genitourinary and reproductive systems. These disorders range from minor herpes to major bladder tumors, from kidney failure to prostate cancer. I have treated men of such great wealth they could buy the hospital in which I did their surgery. I have treated men so poor they couldn't even purchase aspirin. I have treated world-famous celebrities and the people who shine celebrities' shoes. I have treated geniuses and dunces, PhDs and dropouts, men who have read everything and men who cannot read their own names. I have treated the young, middle-aged, and elderly, heterosexuals, homosexuals, bisexuals, transsexuals, and nonsexuals. I have counseled married men, single men, divorced men, and widowers. I have evaluated the promiscuous, the monogamous, and the celibate. All this experience has taught me that, despite the vast differences among them, all men have certain things in common. Three constant observations led directly to this book:

- Men are penis oriented. In the minds of men, the penis reigns supreme.
- Most men (and almost all women) are woefully ignorant about the penis and the male sexual apparatus.
- An alarming percentage of men are plagued by penis weakness or penis insecurity.

Let's look at each of these points separately.

Men Are Penis-Oriented Creatures

Penis oriented means that a man's personality, behavior, and outlook on life are governed in large part by his image of his penis.

The biological and emotional signals sent to a man by his penis make him "penocentric." Usually, the suggestion that a particular man is penis driven contains pejorative connotations. We say things like "His big head is ruled by his little head" or "His brains are in his wiener."

I don't mean "penocentric" pejoratively. I am asserting as a fact the dominance of the penis over a man's being: his self-image, attitude, and behavior. There are extremes—the Don Juans, Casanovas, exhibitionists, and men who are obsessed with sex—but those characters are not the only ones who are penis driven.

What most people don't understand is that all men are penis oriented. This is simply the way nature intended men to be. In many respects, the penis is the organ of a man's essence. It is the axis around which the male body and personality rotate.

The truth of my observation is obvious in our rich heritage of bawdy humor. Is any body part the subject of more jokes than the penis? Much of that humor directly reflects my point about the supremacy of the organ. There is a famous joke about a man who says to his girlfriend, "Women don't have any brains," to which she replies, "That's because we don't have penises to put them in."

Then there is the riddle a female patient once posed to me:

What do you call the superfluous skin around the penis?
Answer: A man.

Or how about the classic story of the mother observing her young son and daughter taking a bath together? When the daughter asks her mother if that "thing" between her brother's legs is his brain, the mother replies, "Not yet!"

Consider the number of nicknames assigned to the penis. Do we have nicknames for arms and legs and livers? Not even buttocks and breasts come close to having the number of monikers we have given the penis. That fact alone is a strong indication of how central the penis is to male identity. Here is a partial list of the many terms for the penis I've heard in my life and in my practice: *apparatus, appendage, bat, battering ram, bone, bone piccolo, cock, dick, dingaling, dong, engine, equipment, gadget, gladius* (a Latin word meaning "sword"; the Latin word *vagina* means "sheath"), *goober, horn, hook, instrument, Johnson, John Thomas, joint, Jolly Roger, machine, manhood, manroot, member, mighty one-eye, one-eyed trouser snake, organ, pecker, peenie, pee pee, peter, pisser, pistol, prick, putz, rod, roger, salami, schlong, schmuck, shaft, thing, third leg, tool, wang, weapon, wee wee, wick, wiener, works, yard, zapper.* And there are probably many more being invented every day!

Individual men, and sometimes their lovers, tag their penises with their own personal and affectionate nicknames. I had a patient whose wife called his penis "Helmut" because its head, the glans, reminded her of a helmet. A college friend called his penis "Winchester" after the rifle. When flower power came into vogue, he dropped that aggressive title in favor of "Mellow Yellow." Famous men with personal penis nicknames include Robin Williams, who used to refer to "Mr. Happy" in his stand-up routines; Lyndon Johnson, who, true to form, called his "Jumbo"; and the King of rock 'n' roll, who referred to his favorite appendage as "Little Elvis."

In a man's psyche, the penis is king. The penis rules its owner as a king governs his citizens. Sometimes, like a potentate who obeys the will of his people, the penis does a man's bidding. Other times, like a dictator, it commands by its own terms and its own rules—rules that men cannot always comprehend. As a monarch, the penis sometimes acts in unpredictable, enigmatic ways. It can be despotic, capricious, and selfish and at other times benevolent, magnanimous, and wise.

When "King Penis" issues a command, a man has little power to disobey. It can turn the mind, the emotions, and the senses into obedient serfs.

Understanding the powerful correlation between the dictates of the penis and the behavior of men in all aspects of life is critical. My father often said, "When it's soft, I'm hard, and when it's hard, I'm soft." What my father really meant is that the penis is an extremely unpredictable creature.

Every wise woman knows that if she wants something from a man, the worst time to ask for it is when he is sexually frustrated. It is far better to ask when he is sexually aroused and his blood has rushed to his loins. His willpower has followed. He will sell his soul for satisfaction. The best time to ask for anything, however, is just after he has had a satisfying orgasm, when his essence has become as soft as his sated member.

On a more abstract level, a powerful connection exists between how men perceive their penises and how they perceive themselves. A man who likes his penis and has confidence in his organ also has trust and confidence in himself. Conversely, a man who distrusts or resents his penis and is insecure about its size or ability to perform tends to have poor self-esteem. It is not clear which comes first, the self-image or the penis image. The relationship between self-esteem and penis power works in both directions. A man who is unsure of himself sexually or has embarrassing sexual experiences (such as premature ejaculation or failure to get an erection) will be shadowed in other aspects of his life by insecurity and self-doubt. A man whose self-regard takes a blow in his professional life may carry that negative feeling into the bedroom. In both of these instances, the penis responds to the realities of self-image.

The penis embodies both the personality and the sexuality of a man. This dynamic can also work in a positive way. If a man satisfies himself and his partner in the evening, he will probably approach his work with self-assurance in the morning; if he comes home from the *board*room with the esteem of his colleagues and the memory of a job well done, he is much more likely to glide boldly and energetically into the *bed*room.

The penis is an extension of the ego, and at the same time, it shapes the ego. The penis receives its marching orders from the brain. At the same time, it dictates to the brain. Sexuality is an essential part of everyone's life. It is the most fundamental human drive, second only to basic survival. This basic truth of human existence deserves open discussion. Sexuality should be celebrated as one of our most valuable gifts. Instead, we either deny it or act as if it were a curse inflicted on us by the devil.

Many men and women suffer both sexually and emotionally. Much of this suffering is a result of a general lack of sex education. In American culture, the issues surrounding sexuality have been barred from public discourse for far too long. This book can help men and women overcome the initial embarrassment, awkwardness, and unfamiliarity of these topics as they come to understand their bodies and themselves.

We Are Tragically Ill-Informed about the Penis

The genitals (and sexuality in general) are still a taboo subject. In an Internet age when pornographic pictures are easier to find than photographs of world leaders and seminude bodies can be seen gyrating on television, the penis still remains closeted behind a curtain of prudishness. Thanks to the candor of the women's movement and the social importance of childbearing, men and women are relatively well informed about women's sexuality. We know the anatomy of the female reproductive system. But when it comes to the penis and its attendant components, both sexes are plagued by ignorance. Only in the last few years have men and women been compelled to face the real issues surrounding the penis and male sexuality. This awareness has been triggered by the increase in public advertisement of male sexual enhancement products such as Viagra, Levitra, and Cialis.

I am always amazed by how little my patients know about their own penises. Middle-aged men are constantly asking me questions that they should have been able to answer as teenagers. They are not only *under*informed but also *mis*informed. The myths I hear about the penis are mind-boggling.

So why is it only now that the real face of male sexuality is starting to be discussed? The genitals are not only the most infrequently viewed of our external organs, they are also seldom even mentioned in man-to-man conversations. Neither joking nor bragging is amenable to the dissemination of accurate information.

The only time teachers mention the penis in classrooms is in attenuated descriptions of how conception takes place. In that context, that mysterious and magnificent organ is reduced to the status of a seed-planter. Most fathers are not much help either. They have "the talk" with their sons only when forced to go through the obligatory facts-of-life ritual. They rush through as if they cannot wait to change the subject to baseball. These brief conversations are usually relegated to some form of the old *Hill Street Blues* line "Be careful out there" or my favorite "Son, you're playing with a loaded gun now!"

Men don't get much help from their doctors either. Pediatricians discuss the penis with adolescents only if they observe a physical abnormality or feel obliged to warn them about pregnancy or sexually transmitted diseases. Nowhere along the line do young men really learn the biological facts. They do not grasp the mental and emotional connection that exists between themselves and their penises. Sadly, it does not get much better when boys become men.

Doctors talk about the penis only when a patient brings the subject up because he has a problem. Even in the context of a general physical examination, physicians will take at most a cursory look at the genitals for signs of gross abnormalities. With older men, doctors might perform the requisite examination of the prostate gland. There might be an item on a questionnaire that asks the patient if he's having problems with his sex drive, usually coupled with an offer to buy Viagra, Cialis, or Levitra. This approach is hardly a suitable entry to a beneficial discussion.

One reason for this reluctance to discuss male sexuality openly is our puritanical heritage. The very word *penis* still has a peculiar shock value. When many people hear it they giggle, blush, or avert their eyes. Certainly, the word perks up people's ears and puts many men on guard, even in a doctor's office.

The other reason men remain ignorant about the penis is that most physicians are undereducated in the area of men's sexual health. Just as with every other organ, doctors learn the penis's basic anatomy and the biological details of what takes place when it performs its various functions.

But doctors (and patients) are taught little about the concept of the *penis mystique*. The penis mystique is that curious realm where the hard data of biology meets the unpredictable and mysterious realm of the mind and emotions.

Doctors should be able to competently answer these questions:

- What makes the penis work and what makes it *not* work?
- Why does the penis seem to have a mind of its own?
- Why does the penis get hard some times and not others?

- Why are some sexual experiences more satisfying than others, even though the exact same reflex action occurs with every orgasm?
- What is normal and what is not?

Men wonder about all of these things, but they are usually too embarrassed to inquire about them. And if they do ask their doctors, they usually get inadequate answers. The truth is that we do not know enough about these issues scientifically. Unfortunately, the psychic realm of the penis is being ignored in medical education, except in psychiatry classes, where the discussion is confined to abnormalities. This is a major problem. If men cannot turn to doctors for this vital information, whom can they ask?

Unfortunately, most men get their most influential penis education from the street corner, locker-room banter, pornography, racy novels, magazines, and images broadcast by the mass media. This is not education. Knowledge of the penis is so central to a man's being—so natural, so normal, and so vital—that we must bring it out of the closet and into the light of day. If we do not, the damaging trend I have observed will continue to grow.

An Epidemic of Penis Weakness

Penis weakness is a major problem for the majority of men. What is most shocking, however, is that it is one of the best-kept secrets in America and probably throughout the world. If my experience as a busy urologist is an accurate gauge, the last twenty years have seen a dramatic rise in both real sexual dysfunction and imagined inadequacy. Far more of the imagined variety exists: huge numbers of men *think* they are deficient in some way, or *assume* there is something wrong with them, or *fear* they are abnormal. Some come to see me specifically to talk about their sexual concerns. Most of my patients come because of other urologic problems—kidney or bladder disorders or prostate conditions—but even they find a way to bring up their penis anxieties.

A patient might have a minor complaint about his penis such as a blemish, an irritation, an itch, or a burning sensation when he urinates. But my experience is that he also has something else on his mind. I can almost predict the moment—as he is putting on his pants or reaching for the exam room doorknob—when he says, "By the way, Doc . . . " and follows with a description of his true concern as though it were a mere afterthought.

What are male patients usually concerned about? It boils down to two categories: size and performance. With all due respect to Dr. Freud, women do not have penis envy; they have penis *curiosity*.

It is *men* who have penis envy. "Is it of normal size, Doc?" they wonder. "Shouldn't it be bigger?" Some even ask if I have a way to make it longer or wider. We'll cover the ever-popular issue of size in chapter 2, "The Truth about Penis Size." The more frequent questions are actually about performance. Performance questions cover three areas: sex drive, erections, and ejaculation.

Older men worry because they seem to have lost their libidos.

Middle-aged men are upset because they used to desire sex as often as they could get it, but now they want to make love only a few times a month.

Even young men are occasionally concerned about their sex drive: "My friends are horny all the time. Sex is all they think about. I'm not the same. Is there something wrong with me?"

Then there are erection worries: "I can't get one"; "It takes me a long time to get hard"; "I can't get it up more than once a night now"; and "I lost it right in the middle of foreplay!"

And, of course, there is ejaculation distress: "I can't come anymore"; "I used to have a big payload, and now it's just a little squirt"; and "My partner complains it takes me forever."

Finally, there is the biggest panic-inducer of all: "My lover says I come too fast."

Some of the questions my patients raise reflect serious medical conditions. Wherever that is even a remote possibility, I treat it as such. A small percentage of sexual dysfunction complaints indicate bona fide medical problems. Most of these cases are older men with organic disorders that impede their ability to achieve an erection adequate for penetration (the classic definition of impotence). A number of physiological conditions can cause impotence. These include arteriosclerosis, diabetes, hormonal disorders, injuries, multiple sclerosis, reactions to medication, substance abuse, and the physical effects of aging.

Physicians have made tremendous advances in the science of diagnosis and treatment of erectile dysfunction. Sophisticated tests can now determine the exact cause of the problem or, equally important, can rule out underlying medical causes.

A varied repertoire of excellent treatments for medical penis weakness is available. These treatments will be described in later chapters. Here it is enough to say that only a small number of patients who complain about their penises have genuine medical conditions.

The majority of complaints I hear daily are expressions of insecurity. They have no medical basis. They are variations on fundamental thoughts of anxiety: "Am I normal, Doc? Am I okay?" In most cases, my answer is unequivocally yes.

I tell my patients that penis power is 1 percent between the legs and 99 percent between the ears. Of course, this is more a figure of speech than a real statistic, but I stand by the spirit of my words— the majority of men have perfectly normal apparatuses. Nothing is wrong with their members physically or anatomically. Whatever problem they have, or *think* they have, originates in their minds. This is the case even if the problem expresses itself in a penis that refuses to obey orders.

Some men have chronic sexual dysfunction that is cause for serious concern. This dysfunction not only affects their personal satisfaction and their self-image but also their relationships and the happiness of their partners. When these problems are rooted in deep psychological conditions due to depression, childhood sexual abuse, or some debilitating inner conflict, they are best served by a qualified psychiatrist or psychotherapist.

Such cases, however, are exceptions. Most men can help themselves with a simple change of behavior and an attitude adjustment. The majority of men who worry about their penises are perturbed because of the erroneous notion that they don't measure up to some (mythological) standard.

When it comes to sexuality, ignorance can be disastrous. The nature of the brain-penis axis is so delicate that a lack of confidence or a fear of failure can easily create a self-fulfilling prophecy. If you *think* you are abnormal, if you are anxious about performing adequately, if you are afraid that your partner might be disappointed, then chances are you have already worried yourself into creating the very problems you fear.

Self-doubt is the biggest enemy of the penis!

This is the vicious cycle: doubt leads to penis weakness, then a bad experience increases a man's self-doubt, and the next time he has sex, his anxiety level is even higher, making the chances of the problem repeating itself greater.

Most men who complain of penis problems are either perfectly normal and don't realize it or are inflating their own difficulties by allowing themselves to get sucked into the quicksand of doubt. I am amazed by how much an injection of simple education and a strong dose of reassurance can do for men who suffer from self-doubt. You will be astonished by what the forthcoming chapters will do for you as we demystify the penis and examine all of the factors that can render it weak.

Why Are We Having This Epidemic Now?

I have witnessed an increased development of penis weakness over the last forty years. It is worth analyzing the social conditions that have created this outbreak. One could argue that men have always struggled with this condition. It could also be argued that the increase in penis weakness in recent years is only because men today feel more comfortable talking about their sexual problems. This is not the case. Powerful social and historical factors have contributed to, and continue to create, penis weakness among men today. Each individual case must have an independent evaluation.

One factor that plays a major role in penis weakness is the increased level of stress found in modern society. Men in today's business world work long hours without enough sleep, exercise, or relaxation. They are often psychologically drained and physically exhausted when they get home. Add financial anxiety, societal pressure, nervousness caused by the rapid-fire pace of modern life, traffic jams, conflicts with bosses, coworkers, or clients, and problems with spouses and children and one can see a picture of conditions that are not conducive to either maximum sexual performance or maximum happiness!

These effects are compounded by the media's highly romanticized image of marriage and family life—an image that creates impossible expectations. Being at your best at anything, especially sex, is difficult when you feel out of sorts physically or your mind is someplace else, preoccupied by other problems.

Few issues have a more chilling effect on sex than anxiety. Stress, tension, and anxiety exact a heavy toll on an intimate relationship. These forces pollute the atmosphere and fill the bedroom with emotional toxins.

Stress has definite medical consequences that work against normal sexual function. During the stress response, blood moves away from the genitals to supply the large muscle groups of the arms and legs. Anxiety, including performance anxiety, can increase the activity of the sympathetic nervous system. Anxiety can boost the flow of norepinephrine, a chemical that constricts blood vessels. This condition is precisely the opposite of what is necessary for an erection—a smooth flow of blood to the penis through open vascular channels.

This problem is compounded when men use alcohol and drugs in an attempt to cope with stress. As Shakespeare wisely observed, alcohol "provokes the desire, but it takes away the performance."[1] The same is true of drugs, including nicotine and prescription medications. The drugging of the American male is a major factor in the decline of penis power. The new craze over "Vitamin V" (Viagra) is hardly the solution.

To men who suffer from penis weakness, the Women's movement, for all its welcome advances, has also contributed to the problem. With increased awareness of female sexuality, female orgasm, and the generally open discussion of women's sexual needs (by way of women's magazines, the Internet, television, and films), men now have the added pressure of having to know all of the intricate secrecies of female sexuality. They are expected to perform with the expertise of a twenty-four-year-old pornography star. For some men, this might not be a problem. Sex in general may still be smooth sailing. For most men, however, sex is an obstacle course— a track filled with snares and hurdles in which one scores points for technique as well as for getting to the finish line. The goal is not just to satisfy yourself, it is also *all* about satisfying your partner. And, in many minds, the man has a responsibility not just to bring a woman to orgasm but to multiple, ecstatic, earth-shattering orgasms. Now that's pressure!

Both men and women expect sexual satisfaction. Partners also have a responsibility to work together through communication and understanding in order to meet one another's expectations and to achieve mutual satisfaction. Every man should cater to his partner's pleasure if for no other reason than to enhance his own. It is important to acknowledge that both genders have been insensitive to the high level of performance anxiety brought on by the new rules. The situation is made even more complicated by the enormous range of variation in female sexuality.

Millions of relationships turn into no-win situations when people aim for some imaginary standard of satisfaction instead of attending to the unique nuances and preferences of their partners. From my clinical observations, the single biggest sexual worry of contemporary men is that they will not provide their partners with orgasms of spectacular quantity and quality. If a man has even one humiliating encounter with a dissatisfied partner, he can succumb to the vicious cycle that begins in self-doubt and ends in penis failure.

The widespread use of vibrators and other sensual aids has further complicated things for men. I have had female patients whose use of vibrators has irritated their urinary tracts. I ask why they continue to use them. Typically, they reply that the vibrator gives them a level of sexual excitement that they never obtain with their husbands or boyfriends. I have even had patients who have become so dependant on their vibrators that they have stopped having sex altogether.

No vibrator has lips, hands, or a tongue. No vibrator can be programmed to hug you when you need to be hugged. But how can a human penis measure up to an inanimate object that is always hard, is always ready to go, never asks for anything in return, and can be totally controlled?

What penis could possibly move like a battery-powered, buzzing vibrator? This issue might be a minor factor in male insecurity today, but it must not be overlooked. My hope is that men will read this book and elevate their sexuality to a level of superpotency, and that vibrators will no longer compete with and replace the actual organ they attempt to replicate.

The main reason for the increase in penis weakness is the way in which men learn about sex. Part of men's confusion is due to a simple lack of accurate information. A teenager came to see me about a minor abrasion on his penis. As I examined him and prescribed a medication, I could tell that he wanted to say something more. Sure enough, he mounted enough courage to tell me that he had sex with a girl the previous weekend and could not ejaculate. He was scared to death. Was there something drastically wrong with him? he wondered. I asked him when his most recent sex had been prior to that experience. About a week earlier, he told me. I asked if he masturbated often. When he got over his initial embarrassment, he admitted that he had treated himself to a veritable orgy of masturbation the day of his embarrassing experience. When I told him that anyone who ejaculates six times in an afternoon might have trouble doing it again two hours later, he was so relieved that I thought he would kiss me.

If this young man did not have the nerve to ask, he might have carried the false feeling of inadequacy into subsequent sexual encounters. This would begin a downward spiral of self-doubt. This happens too often to young men, especially surrounding experiences of lost erections and premature ejaculation. What they do not know is that such events are common among their peers. They happen at some point to every nervous young man. But because they are too self-conscious to mention the subject, they assume that something is wrong with them. In many cases, they remain inhibited for years, if not decades. They avoid sex or approach new experiences with apprehension.

Disappointments due to anxiety are far more likely when a young couple hops into bed without having experienced the old-fashioned waiting period in which couples develop trust and affection. I am not advocating the old conventions. I think casual sex can be terrific when people are knowledgeable, careful, and self-assured. But when the participants are nervous, awkward, and unfamiliar with each other, casual sex can sometimes be traumatic. Unfortunately, a few early traumas can scar a young man for a long time.

The natural bravado of men supersedes their need for accurate information. Teenagers in the locker room or school cafeteria are not likely to hear comments like "Hey, guys, I was making out with Suzie last weekend, and I came in my pants before I even had her blouse off" or "Man, I was just about to do the deed when my dick folded up like an umbrella." Even though incidents like this occur every weekend all over the world, not even best friends confess such humiliations to each other. What an adolescent boy *is* likely to hear are wildly exaggerated or completely imaginary tales of sexual exploits. Those become the standards by which he measures himself.

The situation does not improve once adolescents reach adulthood. Just as much macho posturing exists in bars, golf courses, bleachers, factories, and offices as it does in malls and schoolyards. The result is the widespread myth that a "real man" is ready to get it on any time, any place and knows everything there is to know about sex and women. Such a man never doubts his virility for a minute, is never nervous or scared, and can satisfy without fail any partner who is willing. We don't see the real face of male sexuality; but rather, we see illusions and myths that mask its true form.

This is why most men secretly believe that others enjoy sex more than they do. They further believe that others are a whole lot better at it.

The self-doubt brought on by misinformation and lack of proper penis education becomes magnified by the mass media's obsession with sleek, young, perfectly proportioned bodies. Feminists have made us aware of how insecure women can be when they don't measure up to the idealized images of women in movies, commercials, and magazines. Men are subject to the same insecurities. Those handsome hunks with rippling six-pack stomachs and perfect pectoralis muscles who parade before our eyes in the media present an ideal of masculinity that few men can live up to. It's not just feeling that you won't attract the gorgeous models in the beer commercials, it's what those widely promoted standards of youthful virility do to a man's body image as a whole.

You look in the mirror and see something less than what you see on television or in a magazine, and it chips away at your self-esteem. You think what you see in the mirror is inferior, even abnormal, when in fact what is abnormal is those images on television!

This is not just about vanity—it's about sex. These popular images represent idealized sex objects. Since being a man means being potent and virile, those images are society's models of masculinity. For men, the concept of masculinity has more to do with sex than with anything else. Each little dent in your masculine self-image adds to the sum of doubt that you carry with you to the bedroom. Your penis is part of your body. Your image of your penis, your perception of it, your attitude toward it, and therefore, your sense of yourself as a sexual being, is directly linked to how you view your body.

Another media-related factor is the idealized image of the sex act itself. Sex is one of the few activities in life that we do not learn about by actually watching other people do it. Not *real* people at any rate.

We can peek through the keyhole by watching pornographic films and, a bit more discreetly, mainstream movies. With the aid of our imagination, we can spy on couples in the pages of books. But this is hardly an education in realism. If a man's primary source of sex education is the Internet and pornographic movies and books, he cannot help but get the impression that a "real man" is a sculpted masterpiece with a huge penis that becomes hard as stone on a moment's notice and stays that way, throbbing and thrusting, plunging and pounding, until he and his lover—who is, of course, young, gorgeous, perfectly proportioned, and insatiable—with the perfect timing of synchronized swimmers, have simultaneous, earth-stopping, Richter-registering, shrieking orgasms.

When was the last time you saw ordinary sex on-screen or on the page? What you commonly experience in the privacy of your bedroom is much more typical than the media fantasy model. Even if you had the help of Hollywood scriptwriters, directors, set designers, and special-effects wizards, even if the London Symphony Orchestra accompanied your tryst, you would rarely duplicate what novels and movies tell us sex is supposed to be like.

And what happens when reality doesn't measure up to the imagined ideal?

Men blame themselves. They assume something is wrong with them. They think they are failures. And what is the focal point of their disappointment? Their penises, of course. "What's wrong with it? Why can't it be bigger and harder? Why doesn't it do what the throbbing pistons do on the big screen or in books?"

You might not hear men asking those questions, but I do almost every day. Men think they should have a two-foot-long shaft of solid steel between their legs—a shaft that can pump and pound for hours on end.

That's not a penis. That's a Home Depot pneumatic drill from aisle six!

Most men measure themselves against standards built on fantasy, not reality. They interpret normal, commonplace experiences as signs of personal failure. There is enormous variety among men with respect to sex drive, capacity, preferences, and standards of satisfaction. Yet men assume there is a state of being called "normal." They worry that every little sexual idiosyncrasy they have is a sign of abnormality. Worse, if sex doesn't go as desired, or if they have a disappointing or embarrassing experience, they usually panic. This experience can result in significant self-doubt. Self-doubt creates fear, anxiety, and inhibition. These feelings are bigger obstacles to sexual happiness than having a construction crew in your bedroom (maybe even bigger obstacles than having your mother-in-law in your bedroom!).

Every man I have ever known has, at one time or another, lost an erection or ejaculated sooner than he would have liked.

Every man is, at times, not interested in sex.

Every man has failed to satisfy a partner. Men who take such events in stride know that they are perfectly normal. They march without hesitation to their next sexual encounter.

These are the men who have *penis power*.

A Wake-Up Call

The sad part of this whole picture is that millions of men, as well as their partners, are depriving themselves of full sexual satisfaction.

Nothing is more wonderful than the free and uninhibited expression of sexuality. Nothing is more glorious than the joyful sharing of physical pleasure between two generous, enthusiastic human beings. The current plague of confusion and self-consciousness causes most men to have less sex than they would like. And they enjoy the sex they *do* have a lot less.

Sex should be a fun and relaxing part of life, not a chore. It is life's cheapest luxury. For too many men and women it has become a worrisome task—a source of tension, a burden. It is as if sex is a problem to solve or a test to take. Sex should be a simple, natural pleasure that *erases* worries, tensions, and burdens.

As the product of one of the best medical educations our country can offer, and as a urologist with a busy practice, I want to drive home the message that using your penis for the purpose nature intended is not only one of life's great pleasures, but it is also good for your health in general.

Using your penis is good for your cardiovascular health, your mood, and for your psychological well-being. Penis use is a natural tranquilizer with no bad side effects. Men who are sexually frustrated tend to be tense and irritable. They often seem angry at the world.

Men who are sexually satisfied and feel good about themselves as sexual beings tend to have a positive outlook and a warm glow of health. Sex is also a beneficial physical exercise. Sex is excellent for overall fitness. It benefits circulation, stimulates the nervous system and the prostate gland, and clears up mental "cobwebs" by invigorating the whole body.

Contrary to certain myths, you cannot wear out your penis with sexual activity. There is not a preset allotment of orgasms.

I will sum up my judgment on the vigorous exercise of the penis with the childhood ditty that goes, "Use it, use it, you cannot abuse it, and if you don't, you're gonna lose it."

A word of caution: as a physician who has treated numerous AIDS and HIV patients and who has seen many of them die, I'd be the last person to advise anyone to be carefree in his sexual life.

It *is* sexually dangerous out there. But there is no reason that the tragic AIDS epidemic should inhibit responsible adults who are aware of the risks involved in various practices and who understand what it means to use sound judgment and the necessary means of prevention.

The Secret of Penis Power

The purpose of this book is to help men upgrade the quality of their lives by fully expressing their sexuality. Men have no need to resort to esoteric sexual techniques, aphrodisiacs, or new discoveries about erogenous zones (although it cannot hurt to do a little research into these topics if you're interested).

The real secret to penis power is embodied in a very simple premise:

> If you become absolutely at ease with your penis, the quality of your life will dramatically change for the better.

My goal is to destroy penis weakness in all its forms: chronic or occasional, actual or imagined. My goal is to eliminate self-doubt and inhibition. In the pursuit of this goal, this book will demystify the penis. It will erase all the mythology that surrounds the penis and empower men to enjoy every ounce of pleasure that this wonderful organ was intended to give.

All of this information will help men have a better understanding and greater control in their sexual and romantic relationships. This book will also help women become experts in the nurturing and care of the penises in their lives. It will empower them with the information to understand the men they look to for their own satisfaction.

Used properly, the lessons in this book will help you become superpotent. This does not mean you will have a King Kong–like erection for a week straight. Nor does it imply you will become some stereotypical stud.

I do not define superpotency according to arbitrary standards of frequency, endurance, or technique. Doing so would be self-defeating. It would intimidate men more than they already are and would increase self-doubt and penis weakness.

The concept of *penis power* means achieving maximum enjoyment and satisfaction for both you and your partner, as determined by your own standards, desires, and tastes. *Penis power* means harnessing the full potential of your penis by treating it with all the respect and appreciation it deserves. Learning to do so will do more for your self-esteem than a year's worth of self-help workshops. It will do more for the sorry state of sexual relationships than any talk show, how-to video, or program found on television today.

My message is simple:

- Your penis is as big as you think it is; if you think big, you are big.

- Your penis behaves the way you tell it to, and you can learn how to control it.
- You are as potent as you think you are.
- You are okay, and your penis is okay.

It is important to acknowledge that a minority of men have medical conditions that impede the normal sexual function of their penises. Therefore, you need to be aware of the conditions that may impair your sexual ability as well as other physical factors that can affect your penis. With today's medical advancements, many of these organic penile infirmities can be overcome.

Unless you are one of those exceptions, however, you do not need specialized medical care or intensive psychotherapy.

What you need are facts—a basic lesson in Penis 101. To become the man you want to be, all you require is a change in attitude and some information on how to improve your sexual functioning.

You will find all of that and more in the chapters that follow. By the time you finish this book, you will have what it takes to maximize your penis power. You will live the rest of your life as a superpotent man.

Chapter 2

The Truth about Penis Size

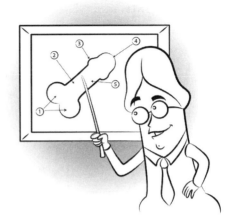

I am constantly amazed at what the average adult does not know about the penis. Most people have a pretty good idea how the heart works, where the lungs and kidneys are located, and what happens to food as it works its way through the digestive system. They even know how babies are born. But nearly half of the human bodies in the world have this odd-looking appendage dangling between their legs, and people know nothing about it. If it were not for that "tail" (the Latin translation of penis), you would not be here reading this page! My patients, both men and women, ask so many elementary questions about the anatomy and functioning of the penis that I am often embarrassed for them.

The irony is that most people are extremely curious about the penis. They have been curious ever since they were old enough to notice that boys have them and girls do not.

For some reason, this natural curiosity is suppressed. As children, we are told it is improper to ask questions about the genitals. We are told that our questions about the genitals and about sex will be answered when we are "older." These questions are seldom answered. Most adults are too self-conscious to seek out the information on their own. If you are reading this book, then I commend your courage and maturity as you come to fully understand the complex and fascinating details of male anatomy and sexuality.

This chapter is a concise, everyday guide to the concerns most people have about the penis.

Looks Are Not Everything

The penis is an odd-looking organ. It has wrinkles and folds and a wriggling network of red and blue vein pathways. Aesthetically, most people, regardless of gender, do *not* find the penis terribly attractive. Some even find it quite ugly.

I am reminded of a remark made by the wife of a fellow urologist. We were talking one day about a case of hypospadias, a rare congenital abnormality in which the urinary opening (meatus) is not in its normal location at the tip of the penis but somewhere down along the shaft. This deformity is often compounded by a fibrous band of tissue known as a chordee. The chordee gives a peculiar downward curvature to the penis.

I asked my colleague's wife if she knew what a hypospadias was. She said, "Yes. That's a penis that's uglier than usual!"

She was a very sophisticated woman who, by her own admission, had seen a significant number of penises prior to marrying a urologist. She was implying, quite simply, that the usual penis is also ugly. Unfortunately, that is a common point of view.

If you were to eavesdrop on women's most intimate conversations, you would seldom hear them talk about gorgeous penises. When they talk about how handsome a man is, they might praise his strong, muscular physique or giggle over his biceps, his legs, or his buttocks. Seldom will they single out his penis as being particularly attractive. Conversely, most men rarely talk about beautiful vaginas. They discuss breasts, legs, and even hair.

When women hoot and holler over male strippers at places like Chippendales, they are reacting to everything *but* the penis. They are really excited by the fabulous bodies of those gyrating hunks and the way the dancers tease them with their *unexposed* penises. The excitement comes from the *possibility* of exposure and from wondering what the penis might look like. If a stripper were to actually expose his member, the thrill would quickly dissipate unless, of course, there was a possibility that it would become erect.

This widespread lack of appreciation for the penis is a shame. I wish the penis were viewed in a more positive light. There is no reason that our genitals should be overcast by a shadow of repugnance or should be deemed inappropriate objects of discussion or admiration.

Nothing is intrinsically ugly about the penis or the vagina. Our cultural perception reflects a conservative and puritanical past with roots in the same traditions that hold sex—and therefore the sexual organs—to be dirty and debased.

It is time for the penis (and the vagina) to be viewed as a beautiful part of the body, and this beauty and its importance should be celebrated and discussed openly. If you cannot find it in yourself to feel that way about *all* genitals, then at least see your own as a beautiful part of *your* body and try to view your partner's with the same perspective. Your attitude toward your penis reflects your general attitude toward sex and the specific way in which you relate to your genitals.

Just as parents see their own children as beautiful regardless of how homely their actual features may be, so too can we look at what has so wrongly been considered a homely and ugly organ and find it lovely to behold.

To some of you macho guys out there, this all may sound a bit "New Agey" or trite. But all machoness aside, I encourage all men to seriously consider the way in which they view their own genitals. A radical change in perspective toward your penis is an integral step toward overcoming self-doubt and self-consciousness. It is equally important for women around the world to muster up the courage and strength to overcome these old and backward points of view regarding the genitals.

The solution is to learn the facts about your body and to develop a new understanding and a new relationship to sexuality and its attendant organs.

Why does this matter? Because just as children who are told they are beautiful think more highly of themselves, a man would feel better about himself—and his sexuality—if he were told that his penis is beautiful. The more beauty your partner sees in your penis, the more *you* will like what you see when you look in the mirror. As a result, you will attribute more good qualities to your penis and bring more confidence into the bedroom. Positive reinforcement is key, and I can assure you most men need as much of it as they can get when it comes to their blessed organ. The mind's eye can turn something with little inherent beauty into something glorious and unique.

If the penis were less concealed, if it were more openly portrayed in art and film, it might come to be better appreciated as an object of aesthetic pleasure. We would come to respect the vast range of differences among penises. In my forty years in medicine, I have seen more male organs than you would see if you filled the Rose Bowl with naked men. I have never seen any two that look quite alike. If nothing else, greater visibility in the arts and in mass media might demystify the penis and might make men less self-conscious about their own. That acceptance, in turn, would raise the overall level of penis power.

One Size Fits All

The appearance of the penis is not so much what concerns men, but rather the size. I cannot count the number of men who have asked me—as if it were just some casual question that happened to occur to them at that moment—if the size of their penis was "normal." No man has ever worried that it might be too big.

This preoccupation with penis size is one of the saddest and most complicated issues I encounter as a urologist. Men compensate for their insecurity with humor or offhand comments. This further distorts the truth.

That is probably why men tell more jokes about penis *size* than anything else. One of the best examples of penis-size humor involves a man playing golf. He hits the ball into the rough. While he is looking for it, he happens to see a pair of tiny feet sticking out of and tangled in some brambles. He hears a little Irish voice calling for help and pulls the little feet out from under the brush. To his surprise, he frees a leprechaun, who, in appreciation, grants him a wish. Without any hesitation, the golfer says, "I want the biggest dick you can give me!" The leprechaun grants his wish, and the man's penis becomes so long that it sticks out of the bottom of his golf pants, drags on the ground, and needs to be tucked into his socks. Overall, it becomes quite a nuisance.

The next time out on the links, the man meets the same leprechaun. "How's it hangin'?" asks the wee one. The man explains his predicament, and the leprechaun, feeling compassionate, grants him another wish.

Without hesitation, the man turns to the leprechaun and says, "Great! Can you make my legs about four inches longer?"

That joke says everything you need to know about what penis size means within the minds of men. The *myth* that size is important is one of the cruelest hoaxes ever perpetrated on mankind. The culture of misinformation has been so deeply embedded in the collective consciousness that men have become extremely sensitive about the length and width of their penises.

There is nothing to worry about because one size fits all!

Your Penis Is Not Too Small

The variation in size among human penises is less than that for hands, fingers, or noses. Penises can be as short as one and a half inches or as long as eight inches. The number of organs that fall at the extremes are exceedingly few. The average length of a penis in its fully flaccid (relaxed, limp, normal) state is about four inches. The overwhelming majority of men fall within centimeters of that average. Penis girth varies less, ranging between one to one-and-a-half inches in diameter when flaccid.

A very tall man might have a longer penis than a short man, just as he will probably have bigger feet and hands. The difference in penis size between two such men will be *far less* than that of their other appendages. A short man's hand might be three full inches shorter than that of a tall man. He might wear a size eight shoe compared to a size thirteen. But his penis might only be a fraction of an inch shorter. I have often seen penises on short men that were as big, or bigger, than those of most professional basketball players.

Of far more importance, given the concerns of most men, is the size of the *erect* penis. The erect penis averages about six inches in length (although most of my patients prefer the phrase "half a foot long"). More importantly, the variation in the size of the erect penis is far less than that of the flaccid penis. If one man's penis is five inches long when soft and another's is three inches long, that two-inch size difference is likely to shrink to near zero when they become erect. It is even possible for the smaller penis to be bigger when erect.

The range in size for erect penises is simply much less than that of flaccid penises. It is as if nature wanted humans to propagate and so made it possible for just about any man, regardless of his overall size, to mate with any woman. So, when you hear men brag that their penises are a foot long, take it with a few grains of salt.

They are either rare exceptions or liars. The only technical way they are not lying is if they are adding to their measurements that portion of the penis we do not normally think about because it is inside the body. (The idea is akin to measuring a hose attached to a sink inside a house because the penis actually begins several inches deep in the pelvic cavity.)

When people ask me about the biggest penis I have ever seen, I tell them it did not belong to any of the oversized professional athletes I have examined, nor to any of the Hollywood "studs" who have come through my office. I tell them that it belonged to a short, slightly built old man who was having prostate surgery. A pleasant, mild-mannered, pious man in his eighties, this patient was married to the same woman his entire adult life. Neither of them had the slightest idea of how relatively huge the penis that had sired their nine children was. I have never had so many helpers in the operating room! Half the nurses in the building wanted to assist me just to view this magnificent organ.

The point is not that men and women are not *interested* in size, but that most wives and lovers do not care that much. Operating room nurses are compelled to look in awe at any huge or anomalous appendage, whether it is a foot, a breast, or even a penis.

Penis Power Is Not Related to Penis Size

Once I assure my patients that their penises are within the normal range, I hammer home this crucial point: *superpotency has nothing to do with the size of your penis*. When a superpotent man makes love, he is totally immersed in the erotic physical sensations, as well as the emotional feelings of intimacy and tenderness. The last thing on his mind, or on the mind of his lover, is the *size* of his penis.

I have seen men with larger-than-average penises who are plagued by sexual dysfunction. I have seen men with relatively small penises who represent the quintessence of superpotency.

I have been dealing with patients and their wives and lovers for many years. I have never had a woman complain to me that her man's penis was too small. It is conceivable that some women make such complaints to their gynecologists or to female physicians. In my experience, a prodigious penis is simply not a priority for the vast majority of women. My female colleagues agree with me.

A much more common complaint is that a lover's penis is *too big*. Intercourse can be painful for a woman whose vagina cannot accommodate a large penis. This is why I have never had one of them request that I make their man's penis longer or wider. They have asked me if I can make it *harder* or perhaps attach it to a more loving and sensitive guy. When women do make a comment about their man's penis, they usually ask me about the feasibility of surgically reducing the size.

There is no such procedure. In the same way, no legitimate and safe procedure to make penises bigger exists. Penile prostheses, which I often implant surgically to treat organic impotence, do not enlarge the penis. They merely fill the vascular compartments (corpora) in the penis with a firm, inert material that makes the penis hard enough for penetration. What the majority of men and women do not understand is that size is determined by heredity.

From my experience, what most women care about above all else is finding a man with whom they have a special and intimate connection. They seek someone who can achieve an erection that can last long enough for mutual satisfaction. The rest of the details are insignificant.

The old homily "It's not how big it is, but how you use it" is one of those penis clichés that holds up to close scrutiny. Many of my women patients complain that their men do not get aroused often enough. They complain that their partners are not imaginative enough. They complain that their penises do not get *hard* enough. One female patient of mine, a true sage, said, "I don't care how long it is. I don't care how fat it is. I don't care how good-looking it is. I just care how *hard* it is!"

What women really care about is the size of your heart and the kindness in your soul. They want good, caring, responsive lovers who are sensitive to their needs and desires. If a woman sees all of these things in her partner, then the physical details, including penis size, become unimportant.

Some women discuss penis size with their friends. Others may fantasize about men with enormous members. It would be wrong for me to claim that some women do not have preferences for certain types of penises. There are women who have certain physical requirements that are necessary for their sexual satisfaction, and there are also some women who are obsessed with penis size. This is a truth that cannot be denied.

Yet the reality of most relationships is that two people who care enough about being with each other will find ways to make their sex lives work so that both parties are satisfied in all aspects of that relationship.

Some of the fascination with large penises can be attributed to the general cultural viewpoint that "bigger is better." The phallus is a symbol of potency, physical strength, and masculinity. It makes sense that, psychologically, some people conclude that bigger penises are better. The fascination with large penises is not unlike men's attraction to large breasts or shapely behinds. Finding someone with those features might enhance the sexual experience because it fulfills a fantasy, not because women with large breasts are better in bed or have more hospitable vaginas. Physiologically and anatomically, what occurs during intercourse has nothing to do with the size of any body part. The orgasm is exactly the same regardless of the physical features of the partner. An experience that may feel different is actually a result of the power of the mind and the emotions.

A woman with an exceptionally large vagina and a man with a very small penis might be sexually incompatible. I knew of such a couple. The woman was nearly a foot taller than the man. They were hopelessly in love but dissatisfied sexually. They believed his penis was the wrong size for her vagina. Through experimentation they learned to adjust their positions and angles during intercourse. They varied their sexual practices so that eventually both of them were more than content.

There are sound physiological reasons why size does not contribute much to satisfaction. Nature, in its wisdom, placed the principal nerve endings that produce sexual pleasure and orgasm right up front. By this grand design, they can be stimulated *regardless of size*.

The man's areas are on the head of the penis (glans), and the woman's are on the clitoris. This means that any penis is capable of satisfying any woman. By experimenting with different positions and by using hands, lips, or even the penis to stimulate the clitoris directly, any man can secure satisfaction for his partner.

Different women are aroused in different ways. I have talked to women who complained that even though their men were endowed with large penises, they were still unable to be satisfied during sex. It is important for any sexually intimate couple to discuss their preferences and to experiment with different positions. Combining penile stimulation with the simultaneous aid of hands and lips is also a great way to help bring a partner to orgasm.

Some of you at this point are probably shaking your heads. I have to ask you, is the issue with penis size truly of a physical nature, or is it the product of a cultural and psychological point of view? I know what kind of penises are out there. I feel safe in saying that most of the issue with penis size is between our ears—in our minds—and not between our legs.

Sex is a unique and intimate experience. Partners who are willing to communicate with each other and work together can learn to compensate for any physical differences.

You Are as Big as You Think You Are

The power of the mind has the most significant influence over sexuality. The only advantage a man with a large penis might have is that he *thinks* he has an advantage. The myth of the importance of penis size is so strong that if a man thinks he is exceptionally big, he might start *acting* big. He might develop such a strong sense of confidence and penis pride early in life that this alone—not the actual size of his penis—might endow him with exceptional penis power.

Far more men think that they are too small. The exact opposite self-fulfilling prophecy takes place for these men. It usually starts at puberty, when boys start to be self-conscious about everything associated with masculinity:

- Am I tall enough?
- Am I strong enough?
- Do I have pubic and underarm hair?
- Is my penis big enough?

Most boys are so insecure that they magnify any sign of inadequacy they perceive. They compare themselves to older boys or men, or to peers who happen to mature faster. They end up convinced they do not measure up. They look down and see a puny, shriveled gherkin, then look across the locker room at someone else's dangling zucchini. They feel inferior.

These feelings of inferiority do not end with adolescence, either. Sometimes they get even worse with age. If men hang around with guys who brag—or more likely, lie—about the size of their erections or tell jokes that leave the impression that a small penis is tantamount to being effeminate, their insecurity may worsen.

Watching pornographic movies makes men's feelings of inadequacy even greater. Whoever produces those films must have an open casting call for men with exceptionally large members. Then all sorts of lighting and camera tricks are used to make them look even bigger.

Many men feel worse about size as they age because they *think* their penises are shrinking. Men start to gain weight, and the added layers of abdominal fat obscure the base of the penis, which used to be visible. Therefore, chubby men may appear to have small penises—especially in their own eyes—because they are looking down over a potbelly. It explains why slim men appear to have big ones. There is no significant difference in size, especially when the penis is erect. In obese men, the shaft of the penis has to traverse two, three, or four inches of prepubic fat from under the pubic bone, where the base of the penis starts, until it is visible.

A man who does not learn the truth about penis size can be adversely affected by thinking his is too small. This sense of inadequacy can persist throughout his adult life. It manifests itself as self-doubt, which can have detrimental effects on his penis behavior. He thinks he is inadequate anatomically, so he must also be inadequate in performance. Of course, that very inadequacy will then be reflected in his behavior.

Think small and you will be small.

Fortunately, the corollary is equally true: *think big and you will be big.* That is the most important thing for a man to know about size. What really matters is the size of your self-esteem and the size of your heart, *not* the size of your penis. Even if it did matter, you couldn't do anything about it. Size is strictly genetically determined. You could pull on your penis day and night, and it would not get longer. You could try hanging weights from it like men in a certain tribe in Uganda, and you might succeed in stretching the suspensory ligaments to the point where it looks longer. But your penis will not be longer when it is erect due to the genetic predetermination of its size, so why take the risk of permanent injury?

The best answer to the question "How big is your penis?" is a firm "Plenty big enough!"

The Big Myth: Penile Enhancement, Phalloplasty, and Penile Enlargement

Every day on the Internet, I get six or more offers on how to make my penis longer, wider, thicker, or more appealing. These ads promise to "satisfy my dreams." They offer me some magic potion or some ridiculous surgery that uses a grafting material that "guarantees" to enlarge my penis.

As my friend Professor Thomas Lue of the University of California, San Francisco (UCSF), a world-class authority on erectile dysfunction, told me, "The surgical 'enlargement' of the penis is no more effective than taking your penis and whacking it with a large wooden mallet, which essentially results in a flattened, squashed, and mangled 'Polish sausage' effect."

There simply is no effective way of enhancing your penis size. The three oral erectile dysfunction drugs currently on the market (Viagra, Cialis, Levitra) only give one a firmer, *but not a bigger*, penis.

One "penis enlargement" surgery that has been foisted on the unsophisticated consumer who is looking to be the "biggest on the block" consists of nothing more than cutting the suspensory ligaments of the penis. When cut, these ligaments, which attach to the undersurface of the pubic bone, give the appearance of length by allowing the penis to hang a bit lower. This effect is produced at the expense of losing the erect "angle of the dangle." Absolutely no length is gained in the erect penis.

The other technique that claims to increase penis length and girth involves applying some grafted material (usually skin, fat, or a synthetic material) within the shaft of the penis. This usually leads to an unsightly deformity. Furthermore, this procedure can cause serious and damaging complications.

There is no legitimate way to increase the length or width of the human penis. From the sincerest depths of my urologic heart, I pity the patient who tries.

I cannot emphasize enough that the unique and individual size of every man's penis is determined at birth by the size of the corpora cavernosum (the two chambers within the shaft of the penis that fill with blood during an erection).

If one thinks of the two corpora cavernosa as "sausage casings," the size of these casings is predetermined by heredity. When filled with blood at the height of stimulation, both the length and the girth of each man's corpora are fixed. Even when surgeons implant a penile prosthesis in a patient with erectile dysfunction, we must custom measure and fit the implant to the exact dimensions of the existing corpora. We cannot insert a larger implant than the genetically predetermined size of the casing (corpora) can accommodate.

When the surgical quacks and adventurists of the world try to stuff the corpora with autologous fat or other grafting material, the result is not only hideous, but it also invariably results in permanent physical impairment.

My advice to the misinformed men out there is do not believe the enlargement and enhancement "bigger is better" ads appearing on the back pages of men's magazines. They are totally illegitimate! Rather, just take a good look in the mirror, gaze down at that friendly organ hanging between your thighs, and be happy with it. If it functions well, then you have nothing to worry about. Do yourself the favor of treating it as a friend. Protect it from the mutilation that will occur if you trust anyone who promises an unobtainable result.

The most pathetic and saddest men I see in my practice are those who have been subjected to phalloplasty (the surgical enhancement of the penis) for the purpose of increasing length or girth. The main problem with any kind of penile grafting or enhancement surgery is that the penis, unlike the breast, is not a static organ. It is quite easy to put an implant in a breast. The breast is one size, remains one size, and does not grow with excitement. The same can be said for nasal surgery, where something can be added, moved, twisted, or upturned because the nose is a static organ.

The penis is quite small and unassuming in its flaccid (resting) state. When aroused, the penis can grow to ten times its resting size! We have not yet discovered a way of implanting a material that will expand and contract and at the same time be physiologically and aesthetically pleasing.

The overwhelming truth is that the issue of penis size is inconsequential in most relationships. The majority of women whom I have interviewed unanimously agree they have no preference in penis size, as long as it is firm and attached to a loving and kind person. The notion that an enormous penis is somehow a sign of manhood or that having a horse-sized member will somehow magically improve your love life is a myth that is propagated without shame throughout the mass media.

If men spent less time worrying about the size of their penises and more time learning how to use what they have more effectively, then all of those hucksters selling the illusion of happiness through penile enlargement would soon find themselves justifiably out of business.

There is, however, one safe and foolproof method for *instant* penile enlargement:

Step 1: Go to your local stationary store.

Step 2: Buy a large magnifying glass.

Step 3: Unwrap it.

Step 4: Hold it over your organ and look down through the glass.

Voila! The Instant Penis Enlarger (IPE)!

Chapter 3

Erection and Ejaculation

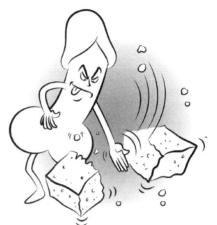

Like a two-headed Hindu god, the penis has the unique characteristic of fulfilling two very necessary roles. It creates life by propelling semen toward fertile ovaries, and it preserves life by expelling toxic substances from the body in the form of urine. Both functions (which cannot take place at the same time, thanks to some very efficient engineering) are carried out through the urethra.

Both functions of the penis are vital. It is interesting to note that, medically speaking, if a man were to lose his penis, he could still urinate, but he could no longer copulate.

Let me dispel two common misconceptions. The penis is not a muscle. The only muscles in the penis are the smooth muscles of the blood vessels. Despite the colloquial term for an erection—the "boner"—there are no bones in the penis. Beneath the skin, which is extremely sensitive (especially the part we call the head or glans, so named because the ancients thought it looked like an acorn), the penis is composed of three cylinders made up of spongy tissue.

One of these cylinders is called the corpus spongiosum. This runs along the bottom of the penis and encircles the urethra. The urethra is a long canal running from the bladder all the way through the penis to the meatus, which is the hole (sometimes humorously referred to as the "eye") at the very tip of the organ. It is through the urethra and out of the meatus that the penis achieves success in both of its jobs.

The other two cylinders run side by side along the upper part of the penis. They consume most of the space inside the organ. These tubular compartments, called the corpora cavernosa, consist of sponge-like tissue filled with blood vessels and tiny chambers called sinusoids.

If you were to look at these corpora through a microscope, you would think you were seeing an aerial view of a delta with its rivers and tributaries. Each tube is surrounded by a tough fibrous sheath (tunica). The tunica joins forces with the interior blood vessels to form an erection. It is the absolute interior volume, limited by the rigid tunica, or coat, that dictates the size of an erect penis.

Erections: Whatever Turns You On

Erections are the result of a complex process that involves the endocrine, muscular, vascular, and neurological systems. All of these systems are affected by psychological and emotional factors. We do not know all the intricate dynamics of *how* erections come and go. We know even less about the all-important brain-penis axis.

We do, however, understand many of the essentials. The penis gets hard in a series of distinct steps. The first reaction occurs when the nerves are stimulated, causing microscopic blood vessels in the corpora to dilate. This is *arousal*.

The factors that excite any given man at any particular time are enormously varied and idiosyncratic. As the pioneering sex researcher Alfred Kinsey wrote, "There is nothing more characteristic of sexual response than the fact that it is not the same in any two individuals."[1] In the more than ten years since *Superpotency* was published, there have been surprisingly few developments in this area. Unfortunately, the "mind" of the penis still remains a mystery.

Whether the stimulation begins with something a man sees, hears, smells, feels, or imagines, it is the brain that determines the level of arousal. The complex neural connections between the brain and the penis are difficult to define and to quantify. The link is so intimate, immediate, and responsive, it is as if the penis has eyes, ears, and a nose. Certainly, it seems that way to an aroused man.

The penis responds most dramatically to *touch*. It is an exquisitely sensitive organ, particularly the glans and the shaft. Exactly what kind of touch will arouse any particular penis is entirely a matter of individual preference, conditioning, and circumstances. Some men like a soft, gentle touch, while others prefer a vigorous, perhaps even rough stroke. Some men respond to the friction of a dry touch, while others favor a moist one. Some find slow, rhythmic movement a turnon, while others go wild over rapid, irregular motion. Some like all of these touches to different degrees at different times.

With the exception of men who have moral or religious objections and those with irrational phobias, I have never met a man who did not respond to oral contact. It is not just the texture of the lips and tongue on the penis, it is not just the psychological charge of having your partner perform such an intimate and generous act, but it is the actual physical effect of sucking. Sucking creates a vacuum. A vacuum creates negative pressure within the corpora, drawing blood into the organ. And that inflow of blood creates an erection.

The penis does not respond to touch only on itself. It perks up when other parts of the body are touched erotically: the thigh, the buttocks, the abdomen, the neck, the lips, and other erogenous zones. Your penis can also get aroused when you touch the right part of someone else's body. As you can see, the penis has an extensive "sense" of touch that is necessary for arousal and also difficult to precisely define.

The penis also has a sense of *smell.* Just ask anyone in the perfume industry! As a young man, I had a particularly memorable sexual encounter with a girl who always wore a perfume with a distinct scent. To this day, whenever I catch a whiff of that brand of perfume, there is not much I can do to keep my pants from bursting at the seams. And it is not just man-made scents to which the penis responds—it is the "perfumes" of nature as well.

Whatever seductive aromas fill the air in springtime, they surely play a role in turning a young man's fancy to love. Many researchers believe that a chemical substance known as a pheromone stimulates the sexual response.

Pheromones are secreted from a woman's skin and vagina. Such pheromones can stimulate a sexual response in males simply through the olfactory sense, the sense of smell. Pheromones are also known to work in the opposite direction. Women can be affected just as much as men by these invisible signals. This natural aphrodisiac is nature's way of ensuring that male and female animals reproduce.

As for the other senses, consider the impact of certain *sounds*: romantic melodies, erotic rhythms, a gentle surf, a breeze rustling through the trees outside the bedroom window. Envision also sweet, erotic words whispered in your ear: "I want you so badly," "You're so sexy," "Do it to me." The penis responds as if it had ears of its own.

Think of the erotic appeal of certain *tastes*. Think moist tropical fruits, ice cubes, ice cream, ice *anything*, and of course your lover's sweat and saliva.

Let's talk about *visual* stimulation. Whether your taste is Frederick's of Hollywood, Victoria's Secret, *Soldier of Fortune, Field and Stream, Playboy* or *Playgirl* magazine, whether it's tight jeans or a diaphanous skirt, a skimpy bikini or a beach towel wrapped around a mystery, your penis responds to what you see. More importantly, it responds to the prospect of what you *might* see.

Arousal involves more than just the senses. The mind and emotions are also crucial players. The same stimuli that may work like magic on one occasion may elicit indifference on another. It all depends on your mood and the psychological undercurrents at that moment.

The strokes, scents, and sights of a person you love, or one you have been lusting after, will produce vastly different effects than the strokes, scents, and sights of someone you cannot stand. Arousal can occur without any help from the senses at all. *Imagination* is often sufficient enough (and is often required).

Just ask any man who has gone through adolescence. That hypersensitive devil is primed to spring forward at the slightest provocation, just like a car alarm that is triggered when someone stands too close.

Tumescence: Stand Up and Be Counted

Whatever the source of arousal may be, what occurs during an erection is a complex physiological reaction involving nerves, muscles, blood vessels, and hormones. When the brain decides it is time for the penis to stand up and be counted, signals travel to the lumbar area (lower back) of the spinal cord. From there, messages are dispatched along a network of nerves to the penis. The tiny muscles within the walls of the penile arteries are ordered to relax. This opens up the corpora channels and allows more blood to flow into the flaccid penis. Blood is *always* flowing into the penis from the rest of the body, but it enters in relatively small amounts. It then flows back out through the veins at a more or less steady pace. Most of the time, the penis stays soft. When you are aroused, however, blood gets pumped to where it is needed, gushing into the penis at six to eight times its normal rate.

The penis then becomes engorged. The arteries distend. The small sinusoids fill up, and the corpora expand like balloons. They press against the tunica in which they are encased. As a result, the penis not only gets bigger, it gets stiffer and more erect. The action is similar to a fire hose that goes from limp and bendable to hard and rigid as it fills with water. Just how big and how rigid the penis becomes depends on how much *potential* volume the corpora were granted by heredity. It also depends on how filled up they become. This, in turn, depends on complex mental and physical factors.

You cannot medically alter the volume of the corpora. This is determined by genetics.

In one of nature's most marvelous and elegant arrangements, the penis *stays* hard because the blood that has flooded into it causes tumescence (the swelling that creates an erection). Once the blood flows in, it does not flow out. Unless the design is impeded by a physical abnormality or a psychological inhibition, the outflow of blood through the venous system is held in check by a valve-like mechanism. This allows the penis to remain hard long enough to accomplish its goal. It is as if the traffic lanes going into a parking lot were widened to allow more cars to enter, but once the cars were in, those lanes were blocked off, preventing the traffic from flowing back out.

When ejaculation occurs, or when arousal is interrupted for some reason (the phone rings, you get nervous, or an unexpected cramp in your leg occurs) the result is detumescence. Detumescence is the release of blood from the corpora. During this process, the smooth muscles around the sinusoids and small arteries contract and the roadblocks in the venous system open up, allowing blood to flow back out. When detumescence occurs, the penis quickly and efficiently becomes flaccid.

Orgasms: Come Again?

Nature designed the mechanism of erection for procreation. The reflex of ejaculation follows erection. Ejaculation is not to be confused with orgasm, even though the two usually, but not always, go together.

Orgasm refers to the intense feeling of pleasure and release felt at the climax of sexual excitement. Orgasm is mainly neurological in nature. It is an electrochemical event centered in areas of the brain that govern pleasure.

In our laboratories, we can trigger an orgasm in animals by stimulating the brain in the right way. Most of the time, men have orgasms when they ejaculate. This is referred to colloquially as "coming."

Most men have had the disconcerting experience of ejaculating without the pleasurable sensation of orgasm. This may have happened when, as adolescents, they were so overwhelmed by excitement and anxiety that they "came" in their pants.

Conversely, some men have experienced the reverse: orgasm without ejaculation. Some esoteric Eastern sex practices can accomplish this. Many of my elderly patients have also experienced it, to their considerable chagrin. This is not uncommon in the elderly age group.

Ejaculation is discharge of semen through the penis. This occurs through a reflex action involving a number of body parts. Let's begin with an explanation of the production of the semen, or ejaculate.

Semen: From Whence It Comes

The sticky, milky-white ejaculate fluid is not produced exclusively in the testicles. It is the contribution of three different organs: the testicles, the seminal vesicles, and the prostate.

The testicles provide the smallest amount of but most important fluid—sperm. In a normal man, anywhere from eighty to six hundred million sperm cells accompany each ejaculation in search of a fertile egg to impregnate. What is most fascinating is that those millions of sperm cells constitute only a miniscule percentage of the total volume of ejaculate.

Sperm travels from each testicle through a pair of tubes called the vas deferens. The sperm is then stored in the seminal vesicles. These vesicles are two pouches that stick out like pennant flags in a stiff wind behind the prostate. They are located near the point where the urethra emerges from the bladder.

There the sperm is mixed with the rest of the seminal fluid, which is a medium to transport the sperm. Some of the fluid is manufactured in the seminal vesicles themselves. The remaining portion is produced in the prostate gland. This gland is an oval-shaped organ about the size of a plum located at the neck of the bladder and surrounding the urethra. Only men have prostates. The prostate not only contributes to the content of the semen but also facilitates the process of ejaculation itself. It helps shut off the flow of urine from the bladder so that semen alone enters the penis.

The complex products of the testicles, prostate, and seminal vesicles form the final composition of the fluid that is ejaculated at the climax of the sex act.

There is, however, another secretion that is actually the first to emerge. That honor belongs to a clear, sticky fluid manufactured in the bulbourethral glands. These glands are called Cowper's glands (named after the seventeenth-century English surgeon William Cowper). The Cowper's glands are about the size of peas and are located just under the prostate.

Small drops of the Cowper's fluid typically appear at the tip of the penis during the arousal stage. Some men confuse this with ejaculate, causing them to panic. They believe that they are ejaculating too quickly. Do not make the mistake of assuming that the fluid contains no sperm cells. This fluid might contain some sperm cells. Only one sperm cell is needed to fertilize an egg. The purpose of the fluid from the Cowper's gland is to help lubricate the vagina. As you can see, this masterfully designed system does not miss a trick.

The Point of No Return

With sufficient stimulation to an erect penis, the reflex action of ejaculation is eventually triggered. The amount of time it takes for this to occur depends on the individual and on the circumstances. The sensation of pleasure involved also may vary with different encounters. A man might experience fireworks and ejaculate very quickly, or he might require an extended period of stimulation in order to achieve climax. The differences in the intensity and pleasure of orgasm are mediated in the brain. These differences entail psychological and emotional factors such as love, romance, fantasy, physical chemistry, and the level of physical and emotional passion that precedes the orgasm.

What takes place *physically* during ejaculation is always the same. This is true with minor variations—whether a man is masturbating in a closet or making love under a tropical waterfall with the partner of his dreams.

When a certain level of excitement is reached, a complex chain of nerve impulses signals the muscles in the pelvic floor to contract. These muscles are located in the perineum, the area between the back of the scrotum and the bottom of the rectum (often referred to as the "'tain't," as in "'tain't in the front and 'tain't in the back"). These contractions close the neck of the bladder and open the ejaculatory ducts. Sperm and seminal fluid can then enter the urethra, where the components are combined.

These pelvic contractions are accompanied by muscle contractions in other parts of the body (such as the lower back and abdomen). They are accompanied by an increase in the heart and respiratory rates, making ejaculation a whole-body phenomenon.

It is at this point, when the contractions of the perineal muscles forcefully start to move the semen on its route through the penis, that men feel the sensations that tell them they are about to ejaculate. From this point on, ejaculation is inevitable. It is a pure reflex that cannot be stopped. Any effort to delay ejaculation has to be made *prior* to this point of no return.

The ejaculate is powerfully propelled from the back of the urethra through the penis and out the tip. It squirts out in several jelly-like clumps, which quickly liquefy into an opaque fluid allowing the sperm to swim to the ovary. Exactly how much is ejaculated varies with factors such as age. The older you get, the less semen is produced. Ejaculation is also influenced by the length of time since the previous ejaculation; the longer it has been since the last ejaculation, the greater the amount of semen. Statistically, the amount of seminal fluid per ejaculate ranges from 2–5 cc (cubic centimeters) and averages about 3 cc, which is about a teaspoon. The volume ejaculated decreases with age because the body simply produces less. The forcefulness of ejaculation also decreases with age due to a natural decline in muscular strength and changes in the vascular system. A young man might project 5 cc of ejaculate halfway across the room while an older man might just dribble a few drops. The mechanism is exactly the same.

It is important to understand that no real correlation exists between the volume of ejaculate and the amount of pleasure that is experienced. Some men actually allow themselves to feel disappointed if they do not produce barrels of the stuff. They mistakenly link their masculinity to the volume of semen they produce.

Some men complain to me that their sex lives are lousy because they do not ejaculate as much as they used to. When I tell them that *everyone* produces less semen as they age and that it has nothing to do with a person's level of sexual pleasure, one of two things happen: they either start enjoying sex again because they are relieved of this self-imposed psychological burden, or they are forced to focus on the *real* problem, which can be anything from a conflict with a partner to a correctable medical condition.

There is a relationship between the strength and duration of the perineal contractions and the intensity of pleasure. I will discuss certain exercises to strengthen the perineal muscles in chapter 15, "How to Become a Superpotent Man."

I must emphasize this important point: any difference in the satisfaction of one ejaculation as compared to another is centered overwhelmingly between your ears, not between your legs or in your perineum.

A particular orgasm might *feel* especially satisfying because of the intensity of the emotions involved or the partner's sexual skills or the circumstances surrounding the experience. It is not because of the volume of seminal fluid. If an orgasm that is accompanied by a large amount of semen *does* feel unusually intense, it is for a good reason. The most likely reason is that the man has gone a long time between ejaculations. The more extended this time gap is, the more fluid builds up in the seminal vesicles. The overdistension of these storage pouches creates the heightened sexual "tension" that is released in an "explosive" orgasm. When you finally ejaculate, you relieve that built-up volume. That is why it feels so good.

The Refractory Period: I Want to Be Alone

As soon as ejaculation is completed, the process is reversed. Heartbeat, blood pressure, and respiratory rate gradually slow down to resting levels. You feel sated and relaxed, and perhaps sleepy.

The scrotum, which reflexively contracts during sexual arousal, and the testes, which rise up within the scrotal sac, relax into their usual positions. The penis, as the blood drains out, reverts to its flaccid state. It is as if the penis, having worked so hard, wants to retreat into solitude and not be seen. The head of the penis becomes extremely sensitive. It does not want to be touched. It does not want to be sucked. It might even burn or hurt if it makes contact with anything. It is as if, after ejaculation, the penis dons a neon sign that reads "Leave me alone!" This is a time of rest. This is a time when the male body restores its energy before it can once again become aroused. This is a refractory period. No amount of stimulation will produce an erection or ejaculation.

Exactly how long it takes for your sexual function to be restored varies considerably from one man to another. Any man will notice distinct variations in his refractory period depending on his partner, the circumstances of the sexual encounter, and other physical factors such as fatigue and general health.

The two main variables that determine the length of the refractory period are age and the length of time since the previous ejaculation. Generally speaking, men need more time to rest the older they are. This means a longer refractory period.

The same man who at nineteen was ready to go five minutes after ejaculating might need an hour at age forty or a full day at age sixty. Conversely, a man who has gone without sex for a long period of time will be restored much more quickly than if he has just ejaculated for the tenth time in two days.

The refractory period is nature's way of making sure men do not waste their energy when they have no semen to contribute. It is during this rest phase that the seminal vesicles are refilled.

These vesicles act like a reservoir with a feedback system. When they are empty, or the volume of seminal fluid is low, the body starts producing more. During that period of time, a man will feel little, if any, desire and will not respond to any efforts to arouse him. As the supply of semen is replenished, the seminal vesicles become distended. When they are filled up with fluid again, seminal production is curtailed. The refractory period is over.

The distended seminal vesicles trigger a neurological signal that produces a sense of "pressure" in the perineum. That is what produces the common feeling of being "frisky." Now that the refractory period is over and the gates are open, the penis perks up, raises its head, and starts calling attention to itself once again.

This is the basic anatomy of erection and ejaculation. Of course, those moments when ejaculation *does not* go right are what all men dread. When the physiology of erection does not operate as expected, men become concerned. This may occur when the mechanism of detumescence occurs at an inopportune time or when ejaculation is untimely. In the following chapter we turn our attention to these very important issues.

Chapter 4

Medical Conditions That Affect Penis Power

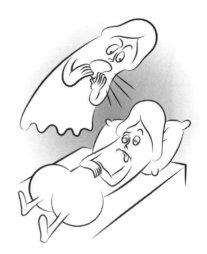

Almost all of the sexual problems that men report to me fall into three basic categories: problems with desire, difficulties with erection, and complications with ejaculation.

Concerns about diminished desire usually come from middle-aged or elderly men who are distressed that they do not crave sex as much as they once did. Concerns about ejaculation present in two ways: too fast (premature ejaculation) or too slow (retarded ejaculation).

"Quick-on-the-trigger" or premature ejaculation complaints are heard mainly from younger men. The "too slow" or retarded ejaculation variety comes from their elders. With rare exceptions, problems with desire that are *not* related to low testosterone levels and certain psychological or emotionally caused ejaculation troubles are not treatable *medical* disorders.

In most instances, these issues are treated by psychological and behavioral therapy. In many cases, those patients who have such complaints do not actually have a problem. They are simply misinformed about what is to be reasonably expected from their bodies.

Years ago, in the heyday of Freud, it was assumed that impotence was a purely psychological problem. Most men who could not obtain satisfactory erections would be psychoanalyzed in order to find the deep, dark roots of their neurosis. Then the medical world learned that erection problems could also be caused by physical disorders.

This significant discovery led doctors to develop sophisticated tools used to distinguish between organic impotence and psychogenic penis weakness. These instruments are particularly useful in identifying erectile dysfunction caused by nonorganic psychological and situational factors. In cases where the cause is clearly physical (i.e., a true medical or biological condition), modern medical technology allows us to make a precise diagnosis and formulate a focused treatment plan.

The reasons that an erection does not occur as desired, or last as long as expected, are even more complex and varied than the reasons for it working properly.

In this chapter, I will focus on medical conditions that affect penis power. We will look at both the organic and inorganic causes of penis weakness in an attempt to reverse the rampant spread of misinformation regarding male sexual health. In so doing, we will eradicate the lack of knowledge of male sexuality.

But first, a few general points are worth considering.

Impotence: "My Friend Has This Problem . . ."

There is no greater symbol of masculinity than an erection. Erection is an anatomical equivalent of wealth, power, and strength. It is "rescuing the damsel in distress," "winning the ball game," "defeating the bad guy in time to save the village," all wrapped into one shaft of flesh and blood. Nothing carries with it more humiliation or self-recrimination than the failure to achieve an erection, a condition known as erectile dysfunction.

Few things are more difficult for a man than admitting he is having an erection problem. Even confessing it to a physician is so embarrassing that men put it off for as long as they can, sometimes until it is too late to correct the situation easily.

Most women have great difficulty in understanding the depths of humiliation a man feels when, in the midst of passionate foreplay, his penis does not get erect. They also have great difficulty understanding the even more humiliating situation when an erect penis suddenly and without warning goes limp.

When a woman's genitalia do not lubricate, she can reach for the K-Y Jelly or her partner can use saliva. Even if she is not terribly aroused, a woman can proceed with intercourse. If she wants to, she can always *pretend* to be passionate.

A man without an erection has no such fallback position. With his penis drooping like a flag on a windless day, he is stripped bare of all pretenses. No artifice can compensate. This is a nightmare worse than dropping a touchdown pass in the end zone or striking out with the bases loaded. Even if it happens just once, the event can be devastating. Very few men are able to shrug it off. When it happens more than once, the shake-up to self-esteem is high on a man's Richter scale. Most men fail to realize that they *should* shrug it off. This happens from time to time to every man.

When a male patient comes into my office and reluctantly admits that he is having problems, the first thing I do is try to make him feel comfortable and safe. He can then speak openly and honestly about his situation.

Usually, the conversation starts with some equivalent of: "Doc, my friend has this problem." Now, we both know who this "friend" really is.

I quickly try to earn his trust and confidence by letting him know that I understand it is *his* predicament, and that no matter what the details of the problem may be, we will straighten everything out.

Once I establish rapport, I take a medical history. The first thing I want to know is whether his problem with erections is of recent origin or if it has been going on for a long time. I then ask if the onset of the problem was sudden or if it was gradual. I ask a series of questions about his personal life, general lifestyle, and emotional state of mind. I follow an algorithm (a preset course of medical questions) in which the patient's answers guide each subsequent question. This leads to an accurate diagnosis. You would be surprised how many men come to me in a complete "penis panic" only to find out that their problem is not medical, but circumstantial. These circumstances include a marriage in jeopardy, aggravation over a business predicament, or just plain mental and physical fatigue.

If my analysis to this point has not revealed any obvious *situational* cause, my line of inquiry turns to medical factors. When the penis fails to perform properly and when psychological factors are ruled out, the diagnosis falls into the clinical category of organic impotence.

Even though only a small number of the men who come to me fall into this category, my first responsibility is to search for a possible medical cause of the problem. Before embarking on a sophisticated *medical* evaluation, I have to be convinced that the patient is, in fact, physically incapable of having an erection. This is often accomplished with one question.

Take the case of a fifty-year-old executive who came to me with a minor irritation on his scrotal skin (the skin covering the testicles). I prescribed a topical ointment. I then listened as this aggressive, no-nonsense mover and shaker gazed at the floor and sheepishly told me the real reason for his visit to my office: "Doc, I just cannot get it up lately."

He said he felt fine otherwise and was not under any exceptional degree of stress. At that moment, my secretary buzzed to tell me that the lab assistant had stopped by to pick up a blood sample. Knowing that this assistant was a beautiful young woman (a frequent occurrence in Los Angeles, where unemployed actresses almost outnumber unemployed urologists), I seized the opportunity to use a visual aid to solve this diagnostic problem.

When the assistant entered the exam area, we exchanged pleasantries. I handed her the sample and she left. I watched as my patient eyed her shapely figure as it swayed out the door. "If she came on to you," I asked, "do you think you would have any problem rising to the occasion?"

"Are you kidding, Doc?" said the patient. "When do we start?"

The patient's "medical" problem was solved because it never really existed! His penis weakness was the result of problems within his marital bedroom, not the result of an anatomic malfunction of his organ. A remark like that does not constitute scientific proof, but in this patient's case, other evidence was in place.

He confessed to having had a recent dalliance with a woman he met on a business trip. During the affair, he performed adequately. From that fact alone, I was certain that the patient was not physically impaired. I counseled him along psychological lines. I suggested that he and his wife might want to see a marriage counselor.

For most patients, the question of whether a penis problem is physical or mental cannot be settled in an interview. I have to use reliable, *objective* criteria.

I have a method that is foolproof.

Fact: all *healthy* males get erections during their sleep. This happens every night without exception. Each episode lasts about half an hour, although the penis is not fully erect the entire time. All healthy men, regardless of age, get these nocturnal erections four or five times a night. They occur in cycles, separated by one to two hours. Most of them coincide with the REM (rapid eye movement) stage of sleep. This is the period during which dreaming occurs. But the erections are not associated with the content of dreams. They are totally nonsexual in nature; even infants have them.

I do not want to create the false impression that a twenty-year-old sleeping penis acts the same as its sixty-year-old counterpart. The total *elapsed time* of nocturnal erections and the *duration* of each erection are age related. They are longest during the teenage years, after which they gradually decline. Normal, healthy men in their eighties still have three or four erections per night. All of this means that, on the average, the penis of a medically fit man is erect more than one hundred minutes a night!

Urologists do not know the purpose of these nocturnal erections or what their function is in the sleep process. Thankfully, they give doctors an important diagnostic tool.

We assume that these nonsexual sleep erections occur by the same mechanisms that cause sexual erections. If a man has normal erections during sleep, we assume he is anatomically and physiologically capable of having good erections during sex. We can then safely conclude that his penis weakness is not rooted in any organic condition; rather, it is psychological in origin.

Conversely, if the patient does *not* have normal sleep erections, we conclude that some organic condition is impeding the process. Our diagnosis is then organic impotence.

If one of my patients happens to wake up in the middle of the night and finds his penis erect, or if he has an erection when he wakes up in the morning (the condition often referred to as "morning wood" or a "piss hard-on" because the morning erection is often accompanied by the need to urinate), he will have the luxury of knowing that his penis is in good working order. Urologists, however, have a more convincing way to make this determination: a diagnostic procedure called the nocturnal penile tumescence (NPT) test.

We will give the patient a simple kit to take home. It consists of a state-of-the-art gadget with loops that look like a small pair of blood pressure cuffs. These are placed around the penis. One is placed at the base and one is placed just under the glans (the head of the penis). Comfortable enough to sleep with, but secure enough not to fall off, the gauges are attached by wire to a meter. The meter is hooked up to a polygraph printer, just like the ones you have seen used in lie detector tests.

If the patient's penis enlarges as it would with a normal nocturnal erection, the pressure inside the cuffs increases. This change registers in graph form on the recording device. We can actually measure the increase in diameter and the degree of rigidity of the penis. We can also measure the frequency and duration of the erections.

This simple device tells me whether a patient is *physically* capable of achieving a satisfactory erection. Regardless of the outcome, my patients invariably feel better because now, at last, the mystery and torment have been solved.

These patients are either relieved to discover that they can, in fact, have an erection and that there is nothing medically wrong, or they are relieved to find out that the problem is physical and not mental. Once I know the problem is physical, I can proceed to evaluate the actual nature of the disorder and outline an appropriate treatment plan.

Before we had sophisticated monitoring devices, I relied on a simple, homemade procedure that can still be used by patients who are intimidated by machines. Take a roll of postage stamps and wrap it around your penis before you go to sleep (keeping in mind the escalating cost of postage). If when you awaken in the morning the perforation between the stamps is torn, there is a good chance you had an erection during the night. The postage stamp test, though scientifically crude, is fairly reliable.

If the patient fails to get an adequate nighttime erection, then it is time for me to proceed with a complete urologic evaluation. Thanks to some remarkable medical advances, physical disorders that used to go undetected can now be diagnosed with relative ease. The men who suffer from them can be treated medically. In the old days, such men might have spent years in psychotherapy while their self-esteem and penis power plummeted to even greater depths.

The key to a successful treatment plan is to obtain an accurate diagnosis, and for most cases, we can determine the cause right in our offices. There are basically three categories of disorders that cause penis failure: neurological, vascular, and hormonal. Organic causes are responsible for a relatively small percentage of erectile dysfunction cases that I encounter in my patients.

The Nerve of It: Neurological Disorders

Some patients are incapable of generating or sustaining an erection because of impairments in the complex network of nerves that make an erection possible. In almost all such cases, the impotence is a symptom of a preexisting neurological disorder. Those disorders are multiple sclerosis, Parkinson's disease, cervical disc disease, and tumors or injuries of the spinal cord. In addition, chronic conditions such as long-term alcoholism and advanced diabetes can lead to damage of the peripheral nerves. This damage can impair erections.

When nocturnal erections do not occur and a patient's medical history reveals any of these disorders, a neurological failure is suspected. To verify this, I sometimes perform a simple exam called the bulbocavernosus reflex test. I insert a gloved finger into the patient's anal sphincter. Then, with my other hand, I gently squeeze the tip of the penis. If the reflex arc is working properly, the anal sphincter will contract firmly against my examining finger. With this simple test, I can determine whether or not the reflex arc necessary for erection is functional.

Fortunately, some of the neurological conditions that cause penis weakness are correctable. If a damaged cervical disc is surgically corrected or a spinal tumor is removed, a patient has a good chance of recovering normal erectile function. Sadly, however, most neurological causes of penis failure are not permanently correctable and are outside the urologist's expertise. With the new developments in the field of erectile dysfunction such as injection therapy, the use of penile prosthetic devices, and especially the safe use of Viagra, Cialis, or Levitra, these organic conditions are often successfully treatable.

When It Cannot Go with the Flow: Vascular Disorders

Of all the *medical* causes of erectile dysfunction, by far the most common are vascular diseases. As we discussed earlier, an erection is in large part a function of blood flow. A lot of problems can be caused by an obstruction in the arteries that bring blood to the penis or by leaks in the venous system that result when the blood in the shaft drains out prematurely.

In other words, if not enough blood enters your penis or not enough blood is held there, your penis cannot stay erect. One of the first things I look for in my patient's medical history is evidence of cardiovascular disease: high blood pressure, chest pain (angina), or pain in the legs after walking or exercising (claudication). These symptoms are all related to conditions that block the blood vessels of your body, and consequently those that serve the penis as well. For that reason, one of the most important things a man who aspires to achieve penis power can do is maintain good cardiovascular fitness through a healthy diet, weight control, and regular exercise.

Through a calculated discussion with a patient, I can get a good idea of whether or not to look further for possible vascular disturbances. In the past, identifying vascular defects in the erection process was extremely difficult. The tests were time-consuming and difficult to perform. They were even more difficult to interpret. All of that has changed. We now have several simple and highly accurate techniques for identifying vascular problems.

A new and especially sophisticated method for identifying arterial insufficiency is the Doppler pulse-wave analysis. This instrument produces an ultrasound beam that we direct toward the blood vessels in the penis. The motion of the blood cells bounces a signal back to the instrument, and the signal responds to the volume of blood flowing through the vessel. The signal is either amplified into an audible sound or recorded as waves onto a chart. The procedure is noninvasive, painless, and extremely precise. Without having to attach gadgets to the penis itself, we can measure the blood flow through individual arteries.

Still more advanced, but more invasive, is a method called penile arteriography. In this process, we inject a dye into the artery that supplies blood to the penis and then monitor the blood flow with x-ray equipment that is sensitive to the dye. This is by far the most accurate way to assess the minute arteries that supply blood to the penis during erection.

However, we do not perform this procedure routinely, since it requires anesthetizing the patient and injecting the dye directly into a very small artery, sometimes producing unwanted complications. In my practice, I reserve this procedure for a few select cases, such as patients with major pelvic injuries or isolated arterial damage that might be amenable to surgical repair.

A Little Prick for a Big Reward: Injectable Drugs

In the early 1980s, a revolutionary technique was introduced with major implications for both the diagnosis and treatment of erectile dysfunction. This technique entails injecting specific vasoactive drugs (i.e., drugs that dilate the penile arteries) into the penis. The drugs dramatically increase blood flow to the penis, usually producing an immediate erection regardless of mental factors. Erection will occur even in the face of significant systemic blood vessel disease.

The most commonly used injectable drugs are papaverine and prostaglandin-E1. In my experience, the injections are the best way to screen for circulatory problems. With one simple injection, we can determine whether the arterial system is intact. The penis either gets hard or it does not. If the injection works, we then carefully instruct the patient in self-administration analogous to a diabetic injecting insulin.

If a patient gets only a partial erection or loses an erection when he changes position, I might also suspect problems with blood flow *out* of the penis—what is known as a venous leak. In some cases, blood flows into the penis normally but is not held in the corpora within the shaft long enough to sustain erection. This usually occurs because the valve mechanism in the veins is not working adequately to trap the blood. New ultrasound technology enables us to diagnose a venous leak easily and effectively.

These harmless and painless methods for measuring the dynamics of penile dysfunction represent medical miracles. Now that we can measure the blood flow through each and every vessel in the penis, we can accurately diagnose blood vessel obstructions and leaks. Even more amazing is that we can take precise steps to correct these problems. In chapter 6, "Blue Pills and Other Medical Cures for Erectile Dysfunction," I will describe in detail the use of papaverine and Prostaglandin-E1 injections to restore declining penis power, especially in aging men.

When Things Are Not Quite Right: Hormonal Disorders

The most common endocrine disease associated with penis failure is diabetes. Diabetes is a syndrome characterized by the abnormal secretion of insulin. Insulin precisely regulates the amount of circulating blood sugar. It is a major cause of generalized arteriosclerosis (hardening of the arteries) and widespread neuropathy, a disorder that destroys nerves throughout the body. With respect to penis power, diabetes is a double threat. It can cause severe damage to the blood vessels as well as the nerves going to the penis.

A significant number of my young diabetic male patients experience a gradual decrease in the *sensitivity* of their penises, as well as a decline in the firmness of their erections. Tragically, many diabetics ultimately become entirely incapable of normal sexual functioning. Not every diabetic is doomed to penis weakness. If the disease is diagnosed early and is properly managed with diet, oral medication, insulin injections, and regular exercise, diabetic men have a good chance of restoring strong penis power—or never having it weaken at all.

Other hormonal conditions can also affect penis power. Abnormal thyroid function, in the form of either an underactive or an overactive thyroid gland, can affect male sexual health. Other potential hormonal problems include the overproduction of the hormone prolactin. This hormone is usually a side effect of certain medications or tumors in the pituitary gland. A deficiency of the male sex hormone testosterone is another hormonal problem. Once diagnosed, these conditions are all easily correctable.

In a moderate number of my patients, a simple blood-screening test might reveal abnormally low levels of the male hormone testosterone. This usually makes itself known by a loss or diminution of sexual drive and desire (libido).

In urologic parlance, testosterone is known as the "desire drug." Most patients who develop this condition have suffered a testicular injury or have had the mumps virus as children.

Mumps can lead to orchitis, an inflammation that causes the testicles to atrophy or deteriorate, rendering them deficient in testosterone production. This condition is also quite common in some of my older male patients. Patients who suffer from atrophy can be treated with either periodic injections of testosterone or the application of a testosterone gel or patch to the skin for transdermal absorption. Both of these methods can bring circulating testosterone up to normal levels in the body and can effectively restore the patient's full penis power. The key to diagnosing and treating these patients is to recognize testicular failure (known as hypogonadism) as the cause. There will be more to discuss on the subject of hypogonadism and the process of andropause (the male equivalent of menopause) in later chapters.

Steroids: Big Biceps and Tiny Testes

It is important for me to emphasize to all of my readers that *there is no legitimate reason to use testosterone if the circulating blood level is already within the normal range.* Contrary to the belief of many of my patients, using testosterone will *not* improve the penis performance of someone whose testosterone level is normal to begin with. More importantly, testosterone and its derivatives, the anabolic steroids, can cause serious side effects. If a man whose testosterone level is within the normal range consumes additional amounts, either orally or by injection, a signal is sent from the pituitary gland in the brain to the testicles to produce *less* of the male hormone. Through a complex feedback mechanism, the body is fine-tuned to maintain just the right amount of circulating testosterone. It can use only so much of it. If you add some from the outside, the body's computer says, "Hey, I'm getting all this extra testosterone—I'd better tell the testicles to stop producing the stuff." The result is testicular atrophy, or "tiny testes."

The widespread use of steroids by competitive athletes and bodybuilders is alarming enough. To realize that some men might take steroids in the vain hope of improving their penis power is even more distressing.

In my practice, I have seen several terrific male specimens—athletes and movie stars with bodies like sculpted marble. They discovered to their horror that steroids were destroying their fertility and their sex lives. Their testicles had shrunk to the size of peas. The results are simply not worth it, even for men whose fortunes depend on their muscular images. For a normal man who is not testosterone deficient, taking anabolic steroids (testosterone or its derivatives) in the hope of turning into a stud is madness.

Do Not Be Sicker Than You Really Are

Any illness can have a dampening effect on a man's penis power. The general weakness and fatigue that accompanies sickness will naturally affect your sex drive and your ability to respond to stimulation. Also, depending on the nature of the affliction and its severity, a patient's range of movement might be limited to the point where he is not able to engage in sex. In many cases, illness brings with it a certain amount of depression or despair, a feeling of inadequacy, and an image of one's body as impaired. All of this can diminish penis power, even if the illness itself does not.

Unfortunately, many sick men give up on themselves as sexual beings because they are convinced they are no longer capable of virile, sexual activities. They might also become unreasonably fearful and refrain from all exertion, including sex-related exercise that could potentially benefit their conditions. Arthritis victims, for example, sometimes abstain from sex because the pain in their joints prevents them from moving around as vigorously as they would like. They are not only depriving themselves of some much-needed and well-deserved joy, but they are also overlooking the significant ways in which sex can improve range of motion and relieve pain as well. My rheumatology colleagues tell me there is evidence that arthritis sufferers can experience relief from pain for up to four to six hours after an orgasm.

Unfortunately, some physicians play into much of the negative mind-set of their injured or sick patients. They advise these patients to limit their sexual activity, or even give it up entirely, when illness strikes. A doctor who goes by the book might even tell a patient that he will never have "normal sex relations" again. What terrible advice to give!

Patients not only get depressed when they hear this, but they also take it to mean that they have to retire their penises and give up all sexual and sensual pleasures entirely. Furthermore, the doctor's negative prognosis is often flawed. Not long ago, physicians told heart patients and people with back pain to avoid exercise. Today, we prescribe exercise programs for their rehabilitation and advise against being sedentary. In many cases, the same is true of sex. I advise and encourage my patients to use their penises to bring cheer to the sickbed, rather than allowing the penis to shrivel up before its time.

If your doctor tells you to abstain from exercising your penis power, get a second opinion! He or she may be misinformed or may simply be old-fashioned. Illness might *limit* your sexuality, but it does not have to *eliminate* it. For most individuals, the solution involves simply learning new habits. Your condition might mean that you take longer to achieve an erection, in which case you can learn to be more patient and your partner can learn new ways to stimulate you.

Your illness might make it impossible to make love in the positions to which you are accustomed. If so, practice the ones that do work. You might have to have sex less often or less vigorously, but instead of lamenting that situation, you can learn to fully savor the slow and gentle sensuality that you used to hurry through.

If you have intercourse less often, you might be able to enjoy oral sex or mutual masturbation *more* often. Such changes make sex different, not inferior. They should be viewed as opportunities for new experiences, rather than reasons to feel sorry for yourself or to give up one of life's greatest pleasures.

Prescription Medications: Is the Pharmacist Really Your Enemy?

A television producer that I had treated for a urinary infection came to see me. The minute I walked into the examining room, I could tell from his facial expression that he had not come to see me only about the infection. Whatever was on his mind was serious, and not something he found easy to talk about. When he finally said, "Doctor, I cannot get hard anymore," I was shocked. He had a reputation as a Casanova of note. He took great pride in his penis power.

We talked for a while about what was going on in his life. I explored the possibility that he, as a single man who liked a variety of partners, might feel frightened by the AIDS epidemic. He rejected that, stating he was careful to sleep with thoroughly screened partners and always practiced safe sex. I thought he might be under some stress or physical strain given the demands of his profession. He assured me that his life was no more pressured than before, when he had no penis problems. In fact, he loved to use sex as an outlet for his built-up tension. His recent sexual failures were unprecedented. He could not figure out what had happened.

When I took his medical history in preparation for a complete examination, I stumbled upon the answer. Since I had last seen him, he had been diagnosed with high blood pressure. Being well aware of the effects of hypertension on penis power, I knew exactly what the problem was. The good news was that the hypertension itself was not affecting his penis power. The bad news, however, was that the prescription medication he was taking to control it *was* having an effect on his penis power.

A number of therapeutic drugs can cause erection or ejaculation problems, even in men with excellent penis attitudes. Unfortunately, very few rigorous scientific studies have been performed on the subject, so most of what we know about penis weakness that is associated with the use of common medicines is anecdotal or reported by manufacturers as possible side effects.

When I suspect that a drug might be responsible for a patient's problem, I do an informal test. This test consists of reducing the dosage or eliminating the drug entirely to see if the patient's penis power is restored. This is done with the cooperation of the primary physician and with all possible safeguards observed. In the case of the television producer, it was not long after we safely lowered the dosage of his antihypertensive medicine before he was back to his old tricks.

Blood pressure medications are not the only culprits, although they are probably the most common. If you were to peruse the *Physician's Desk Reference* (the bible of drug side effects), you would see that sexual dysfunction is listed as a potential side effect of virtually every antihypertensive agent.

These medications work in different ways to lower blood pressure, so their effects on the penis also vary. If you are taking medication for high blood pressure and suspect that it may be adversely affecting your penis power, then you should consult your physician. You might be able to switch to a class of drugs whose ingredients will not keep you from being a superpotent man.

Other drugs that can diminish penis power include some medications used to increase the output of urine. These drugs are known as diuretics. In addition, certain medications used to treat anxiety, depression, and other psychiatric disturbances can cause diminished libido, retarded ejaculation, or erection problems. Various ulcer medications can also cause impotency in some patients because they disrupt the production of testosterone.

I must caution anyone taking prescription medications not to arbitrarily give them up or alter their dosages. If you suspect that a prescription drug is negatively affecting your penis power, be sure to consult with your physician before doing anything on your own. Reducing a dosage or stopping the use of a particular medication can cause an extremely complicated and potentially life-threatening situation. Even a well-trained physician is not always able to tell with certainty whether a specific medication is causing the problem. Many forces might be contributing to your inability to get an erection, not just the medication. Most patients who take such drugs (i.e., hypertension medication) are of advanced age, may suffer from more than one illness, may take a variety of medications, and may have other habits that could be adversely affecting their penis power.

More important are the underlying effects of the disease itself. High blood pressure alone can weaken penis power. Approximately 10 percent of patients who require antihypertensive drugs have significant penis weakness *before* starting treatment.

Similarly, depression triggered by the illness itself can also cause sexual dysfunction. How can we be certain whether it is the disease, the drug, the psychological effects of the sickness, or a combination of all of the above? The sexual side effects of the drugs have to be weighed against the consequences of the diseases themselves. In some cases, switching medications or adjusting the dosage is an easy solution. However, when that is not possible, it might be wiser to live with diminished penis power than to risk aggravating a serious medical condition by disrupting its treatment.

Such decisions require delicate clinical judgment, which is why it is important to have a frank and thorough discussion with your physician and commit to a rigorous scrutiny of all possible options. The point to take away from this section is do not throw your prescription medications down the toilet in the quest for a firmer erection at the risk of a stroke, heart attack, or even death. Quite simply, "It ain't worth it!"

It's Not All Fun and Games: Recreational Drugs

Scenarios such as the one with the television producer have been repeated many times in my office. These events occur not only with prescription drugs, but also with so-called recreational substances.

Drug and alcohol abuse and addiction can cause everything from temporary penis failure to long-term impotence. Some substances create the *illusion* of enhanced sexuality because they seem to take the edge off, calm you down, lower inhibitions, and produce a heightened sensitivity. To paraphrase one of Shakespeare's wisest observations: drugs might add to desire, but they just as equally take away from performance.

"Candy is dandy, but liquor is quicker" is a common expression. We all know the routine. You have a few drinks, and everything from your tongue to your toes loosens up. Wallflowers start to dance, the tongue-tied become candid and verbose, and the sexually repressed become Lotharios.

If the object of your attention has also been drinking, suddenly anything and everything becomes possible. For those reasons, alcohol has become as much a part of lovemaking for some people as soft lights. There is nothing dangerous about moderate, judicious drinking. If the moderate consumption of alcohol reduces anxiety, slows you down, and delays ejaculation a bit, then alcohol can be a boon to penis power.

Unfortunately, alcohol can also be the greatest enemy of your penis. If you overdo it, your penis will poop out when it ought to pop out.

More significant to our discussion are the effects of alcohol *abuse*. Overdoing it with alcohol or illicit substances makes it more difficult to become aroused. Overindulgence delays ejaculation, reduces the pleasure and intensity of orgasms, and greatly diminishes penis rigidity (firmness of erection).

In my practice, nearly 50 percent of the chronic alcoholics I have counseled experience either total or partial impotence. The short-term effects appear to be based on alcohol's sedative action on the central nervous system. The long-term or chronic effects include severe nerve damage of the kind that can diminish penis sensitivity and permanently impair the ability to get an erection.

Many patients have told me that marijuana enhances their penis power. Some studies have indicated that marijuana can, in fact, slow the ejaculatory process. In other words, an erection can be maintained for a longer period of time before orgasm. For a younger man who might be quick on the trigger, this can be perceived as "enhanced" potency because marijuana might lower inhibitory mechanisms, reduce anxiety, and heighten erotic sensations.

I must recommend extreme caution about jumping to the conclusion that marijuana is an aphrodisiac or an aid to penis power. Since marijuana is a mind-altering substance, its effect on sexuality is most likely illusory. Research shows that the negative effects of marijuana are similar to those of alcohol. Therefore, I suspect that, like alcohol, it would be hostile to penis power in the long run. There is good evidence that long-term marijuana smoking weakens overall fitness and reduces energy and motivation. Such effects would not bode well for a superpotent man.

In addition to alcohol and marijuana, cocaine can be detrimental to penis power. When Cole Porter wrote that he doesn't get a kick from cocaine, he might not have been thinking about sex. But the message applies: where penis power is concerned, cocaine is certainly no kick. In the short term, cocaine has an excitatory effect on the nervous system. It can stimulate arousal and make every sensory experience *seem* more intense. In the long run, cocaine will turn a superpotent man into a super-*wimp*.

Pharmacologically, cocaine decreases the reuptake of the neurotransmitter catecholamine. This chemical is essential for the adequate completion of the erection process. Failure to get and maintain erections is a common complaint from cocaine abusers. No man who aspires to penis power should go anywhere near this drug. As for other illicit drugs such as amphetamines or ecstasy, no superpotent man should ever use them.

As for amphetamines, let me remind you of the 1960s poster that said, "Speed kills!" Well, it certainly kills libido, ejaculatory function, and erections. Its long-term sexual impact is devastating. This is also true for drugs in the narcotic family such as heroin, codeine, Demerol, and pain killers (i.e., Vicodin, Valium, Oxycontin). Users of these drugs experience a drastic reduction in libido, as well as chronic difficulty with erections. Unquestionably, these recreational drugs produce the antithesis of penis power—penis failure.

One more drug must be mentioned, especially since it has long been associated with mating rituals—nicotine. As if there were not enough reasons to stop smoking (or never start), consider this: smoking has been linked to penis weakness.

Several studies have demonstrated that cigarette smoking is more prevalent among impotent men. In another study, animals exposed to tobacco smoke or intravenous nicotine were unable to produce or maintain erections.

There is a simple scientific reason for this. Nicotine constricts blood vessels. When you smoke, the supply of arterial blood to the penis is reduced, making it more difficult to get a firm erection. Simply put, smoking is as bad for your penis as it is for your lungs. If you want to be a man of penis power, just say no to drugs and nicotine.

Premature Ejaculation

Premature ejaculation (PE) is one of the most common forms of sexual dysfunction in men today. Even though it has been established that premature ejaculation is a prominent male sexual disorder, the true cause and frequency of PE remain unknown.

PE affects more than 30 percent of the male population and is consistent across all age groups. It is, however, more common in my younger patients. Unlike erectile dysfunction, which increases with age, the likelihood of premature ejaculation is generally not affected by age, marital status, race, or ethnicity. Some men face this problem from adolescence through adulthood.

PE has historically been perceived as a sexual dysfunction of psychological versus organic origin. Only within the past decade or so have organic etiologies of PE been explored.

PE is a nuisance that many men do not realize they can fix. There are a number of self-help techniques recommended by sexual therapists and urologists that have proven to be very effective for men who suffer from PE. Recently, there has also been significant research into the development of "off-label" pharmacological therapies that can help delay ejaculation.

Unfortunately, there is no oral or topical medication currently approved by the Food and Drug Administration (FDA) for premature ejaculation. However, a number of therapies that are still in the testing phase have shown varying degrees of success.

According to the American Urological Association, there are as many as five definitions for premature ejaculation that urologists use to assess a patient with PE. A substantial amount of agreement exists among the various definitions.

These definitions state that premature ejaculation is the inability to control ejaculation sufficiently for both partners to enjoy sexual interaction. It is usually marked by a persistent or recurrent onset of orgasm and ejaculation with minimal stimulation before, on, or shortly after penetration. It occurs before the person wishes to ejaculate. This is usually compounded by distress and frustration within a sexual relationship.

Premature ejaculation is not life-threatening. The main issue with premature ejaculation is its impact on the quality of life for those who suffer from its effects. In a recent survey of men with and without PE, 90 percent of those surveyed ranked fulfilling a partner's sexual needs as very or extremely important.

Men who have a problem with premature ejaculation find that it is increasingly difficult to satisfy their partners through intercourse. Their partners feel increasingly frustrated. This scenario creates a negative chain reaction. Coupled with poor communication and a lack of awareness, PE can cause severe rifts in an otherwise healthy, intimate relationship.

Men who suffer from PE can have a diminished sense of self-esteem and increased anxiety because of the recurring embarrassment associated with PE. For the partners of those men, it can also be a very frustrating problem. If a couple does not *communicate* openly about PE, it can lead to distress and dissatisfaction within the relationship, mistrust, and resentment between two partners.

If You Need Help, Come and Get It

Surprisingly, less than 20 percent of men with premature ejaculation seek treatment. In my practice, I find the most common barriers to seeking treatment are the embarrassment over one's inability to control ejaculation and the reluctance to admit the problem exists. The public has the misperception that PE is *transient* and solely psychological. Add to that the lack of knowledge regarding the availability of pharmacological therapies and the common confusion regarding the difference between erectile dysfunction (ED) and premature ejaculation (PE), and it is no wonder that PE remains, for the most part, a hidden problem. This is truly a sad predicament for some men.

To fully understand what is happening in men who experience premature ejaculation, it is important to look at the normal physiology of male sexual response. As we discussed in our analysis of erectile dysfunction, achieving a normal erection is a complex event. Erection involves vascular and neurological phenomena with hormonal and psychological influences. Abnormalities in any of these areas can lead to erectile or ejaculatory dysfunction.

Ejaculation and erection usually occur together, even though they are not regulated by the same mechanisms, and one can occur without the other. During each sexual act, ejaculation is initially under some control until one reaches that level of excitation we call the point of "ejaculatory inevitability." This is the point when ejaculation becomes completely reflexive and out of one's control.

Interestingly, the "sensation" that occurs with orgasm is not reflexive. Orgasm is a distinct cognitive and emotional event. Remember that normal male sexual response follows a cycle with four phases: excitement (desire), plateau (arousal), ejaculation and orgasm, and a resolution phase, which involves a refractory period. During the refractory period, a man cannot ejaculate again. Although the cause of premature ejaculation remains largely unknown, it is believed that the sexual response cycle in men with PE involves a disruption of the normal curve of ejaculatory response. This is usually characterized by a steep excitement phase with a shortened plateau phase leading to premature ejaculation and a rapid resolution phase.

Anxiety also appears to play an important role in PE. Anxiety activates the sympathetic nervous system and lowers the ejaculatory threshold.

I see problematic premature ejaculation in my patients who are sexually inexperienced or in those men who have a poor understanding of the sexual response cycle, infrequent sex, or problematic relationships. To put this whole picture into numbers, the average length of intercourse for men with PE is under two minutes. For men with normal ejaculatory response, it is somewhere between seven and a half and nine minutes. Don't we all wish it were longer?

If you are concerned that you may be suffering from premature ejaculation, ask yourself the following questions:

- Are you dissatisfied with your sex life because of your lack of staying power?
- During the majority of times you have sex, do you ejaculate before you wish?

If you answered yes to these questions, or if you identify with the time comparison mentioned and PE is a problem for you, there are solutions available. Urologists, unlike most others in the health-care community, are becoming more equipped and better informed to help patients deal with this ever-present problem. We have the expertise to make available a wide variety of topical and oral "off-label" agents that can be used to prolong your staying power.

Off the Record

Some of my patients try self-help approaches prior to seeking counseling or pharmacotherapy for PE. These techniques include precoital masturbation, the utilization of multiple condoms, or the use of desensitizing creams to reduce penile sensitivity. They also include engaging in distraction techniques (mental exercises) during foreplay and intercourse and aggressive thrusting during intercourse to speed their partner's satisfaction.

Many of these techniques, however, can actually exacerbate PE. They help the patient deliberately ignore the sexual sensations needed to establish ejaculatory control.

Currently, there are several pharmacological strategies used "off label" for the treatment of PE. These include topical local anesthetics, PDE-5 inhibitors (i.e., Viagra, Levitra, or Cialis), and the "chronic" (daily or regular) use of a class of drugs designed to treat depression called selective serotonin reuptake inhibitors (SSRIs). These drugs can be taken either daily or on demand.

The goals of these treatments are similar to the self-help treatments: the objective is to extend the plateau period and delay ejaculation, which affords the patient greater control over his ejaculation. This ultimately leads to greater sexual satisfaction for both the patient and his partner.

SSRIs were initially formulated for continuous daily use to treat depression. Surprisingly, many patients noted the retardation or delay of ejaculation while taking these drugs. Of the SSRIs, the most commonly used are Paxil, Prozac, and the tricyclic antidepressant Anafranil.

Each of these drugs is effective in delaying ejaculation, but Paxil has been found to exert the greatest effect. Unfortunately, the optimal dose at present for the management of PE remains unclear, although it has been found that chronic use is more effective than on-demand dosing.

In my experience, combining Paxil with some of the PDE-5 inhibitors (i.e., Viagra, Levitra, Cialis) has an even higher success rate. Recently, a medicine called Priligy (dapoxetine) was developed specifically for the management of premature ejaculation. It is rapidly absorbed and increases ejaculatory delay from the first dose. Dapoxetine is administered on an "as needed" basis. This drug significantly increases patient control over ejaculation. This results in an increase in patient and partner satisfaction. Although Priligy is still waiting for approval by the FDA, its future looks promising in resolving the problem of premature ejaculation.

A History of Treating PE

Prior to 1990, when urologists began trying the off-label use of a number of these antidepressants to treat PE, psychotherapy was considered the treatment of choice. The problem was viewed as a psychological impasse and not a physical failure. In the 1940s, clinicians proposed the "stop start" technique, also known as the Masters and Johnson method. This method involves stopping intercourse when the man perceives ejaculatory inevitability, allowing it to subside, and then resuming intercourse, repeating this cycle until both partners are satisfied. In the late 1960s, sexual therapists developed a model that included individual and joint therapy sessions, along with behavioral techniques such as the "sensate focus" and the "squeeze" technique. With this technique, the man or his partner firmly squeezes the glans (tip or head of the penis) prior to ejaculatory inevitability. One can also squeeze the base of the penis, which constricts the flow of ejaculate in addition to pushing blood out of the penis in order to reduce an erection. Both of these versions of the "squeeze" method essentially force a delay of ejaculation. Each of these techniques, or some combination thereof, has proven to be very helpful for men who have PE. You can find out more about these techniques in chapter 15, "How to Become a Superpotent Man."

I recommend to my patients that they first try these nonpharmacological self-help techniques. If they still report difficulty in delaying ejaculation, I may recommend one of the "off-label" uses of SSRIs or PDE-5 inhibitors mentioned earlier.

Men should realize that premature ejaculation can be overcome. It should be viewed as simply another challenge in the quest to becoming a superpotent man. I have known many superpotent men who overcame PE and have gone on to have healthy and long-lasting intimate relationships.

The only question is whether you are willing to over*come* what makes you *come* too quickly.

Chapter 5

Prostatic and Other Urologic Diseases

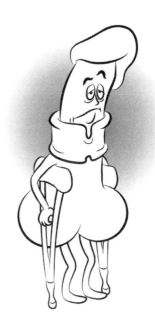

As if getting old is not difficult enough, a significant number of aging men develop a very frustrating and sometimes painful condition known as benign enlargement of the prostate, or benign prostate hypertrophy (BPH).

BPH: Don't Panic!

BPH is present in more than half of all men over the age of fifty. BPH is known for creating an obstruction to the flow of urine. BPH is not related to prostate cancer, so do not panic!

Prostate cancer can be life-threatening, whereas BPH is a benign condition that causes discomfort, incomplete bladder emptying, frequent urination (particularly at night), and a weak urinary flow. BPH is not lethal, but it certainly carries symptoms that affect the quality of daily life. BPH can best be described by this anecdote, told to me by a patient a number of years ago:

> A patient walks into a urologist's office and sits down in the consultation room. The doctor, who has a stutter, asks the patient, "What is is is is wr-wr-wr-wrong wi-wi-with ya-ya-you?" The patient answers, "Well, Doc, I piss the way you talk."

Now, let's take a look at a particular case that will help shed light on the issues related to prostate disease.

Jerry was a sixty-six-year-old chemistry professor who came to see me because he was having difficulty urinating. He was waking up three or four times a night to urinate. His urine flow was slow and irregular. He felt a sensation of incomplete bladder emptying. All of these complaints suggested he might be suffering from a benign enlargement of his prostate.

Look at the prostate as a collar or a doughnut surrounding the neck of the bladder, and look at the bladder as an upside-down balloon. As a man gets older, the collar or doughnut (prostate) tends to get bigger and the hole in the doughnut smaller. The shrinking hole pinches the neck of the bladder, making it more difficult to urinate. This causes the bladder to work harder to empty itself. This phenomenon can lead to other symptoms besides the ones Jerry reported. These symptoms may be blood in the urine, a dribbling urinary stream, painful urination, occasional incontinence, and sometimes pain in the lower back, pelvis, or lower abdomen.

I took a detailed medical history from Jerry, after which I performed a digital rectal examination (DRE) with my "educated" gloved finger. I assessed the size and consistency of his prostate. I then used a funnel-like device that measures the urinary flow rate. I performed a bladder scan to assess Jerry's residual urine, trying to determine his ability to completely or incompletely empty his bladder. Next, I performed a quick prostatic ultrasound. This test projects sound waves through the prostate to search for signs of cancer. Fortunately, this test turned out to be negative.

Finally, I used a cystoscope, a fiberoptic instrument that is inserted directly into the urinary channel. With the help of various lenses, doctors can examine the entire length of the urethra. They can look directly at the prostate and then into the bladder. The instrument enables them to check for tumors, polyps, stones, and other causes of irritation. In addition, it allows them to assess the size and degree of prostatic obstruction.

Like most patients, Jerry was alarmed when I told him I wanted to use the cystoscope. "You're going to stick what in where?" he gasped. I assured him there would be no harm and minimal discomfort. This procedure, when skillfully performed, is relatively painless and is done in the office in about thirty seconds. I told him that if we hurt him at all, there would be no charge—a promise I make without hesitation—and believe me, I do not like to work for free!

Following this complete examination, I concluded that Jerry's prostate was enlarged to the point where damage might eventually be done to his bladder or his kidneys. I recommended aggressive treatment to reduce the degree of prostate obstruction in the form of a surgical procedure known as a prostatectomy.

Jerry panicked. He started sweating heavily and stammering. He was panicked not because of the possibility of surgery and not because he did not trust me to perform the surgery (which I had done successfully on thousands of patients, including Jerry's older brother *and* his uncle), but because he thought that the operation would render him a penis weakling. Jerry's reaction is so common among men with prostate disease—indeed with any kind of problem in the pelvic area—that I must state emphatically,

> Prostatectomy, when done for benign disease, does not cause impotence or any loss of penis power!

Alternatives to a Prostatectomy

Over the past several years, many excellent nonsurgical treatments for BPH have been developed. These treatments have proven to be very effective, noninvasive, and safe. They can be completed with minimal side effects.

In the realm of medication, two drugs in particular act directly to stop and even reverse enlargement of the prostate gland. The older of these two drugs, Proscar (finasteride), reduces a potent androgen (the male hormone equivalent to the female estrogen) that is responsible for the enlargement of the prostate. Although this drug works slowly over time, most urologists note a reduction in both the overall size of the prostate and the severity of obstructive symptoms. The only drawback to the drug is that since it reduces the blood concentration of a potent androgen, it can, on occasion, affect the patient's libido.

A newer drug, Avodart (dutasteride), also improves the symptoms of prostatic enlargement. This drug reduces the androgen that is responsible for prostatic enlargement. It also reduces the risk of acute urinary retention and the need for BPH-related surgery. Over the course of many months, my patients have reported impressive reductions in the symptoms of prostatic obstruction with the use of Avodart, and also minimal side effects.

I often prescribe three other drugs along with Avodart or Proscar. These drugs operate by an entirely different mechanism of action.

These drugs (Flomax, Rapaflo, and Uroxatrol) are known pharmacologically as alpha-blockers. To give a visual representation as to how they work, we return to the analogy of the bladder as an upside-down balloon and the prostate as a doughnut or collar around the neck of the balloon. When men get older, the doughnut gets bigger and the hole in the doughnut gets smaller. The alpha-blockers make the hole in the doughnut (the prostate) bigger. This allows a more complete emptying of the bladder. When alpha-blockers are taken at the same time as anti-androgens (Proscar or Avodart), they work synergistically, and symptoms of benign enlargement of the prostate can often be dramatically improved without surgery.

Turn Up the Heat: TUMT

Not all men with symptoms of BPH respond well to these drugs. In some cases, the degree of prostatic obstruction is so pronounced that a more aggressive approach is needed.

With today's advancements in treatment, even these more serious cases can be handled without surgery. A nonsurgical treatment for BPH was developed a number of years ago. This treatment involves the use of heat in the form of microwaves. The treatment is known as dose-optimized thermal therapy (DOT), or transurethral microwave therapy (TUMT). This technique delivers a specific "best dose" of heat to a patient's prostate, reducing the obstructive element and allowing the maximum relief of symptoms with the fewest side effects.

To be certain that the patient is a good candidate for thermal therapy and the DOT or TUMT procedure, I perform a thorough evaluation of the patient prior to making any decisions. I first evaluate the patient with the cystoscope, as well as with a prostate ultrasound. The ultrasound is used to assess both the size of the prostate and the degree of obstruction. If the degree of prostatic obstruction is significant, the patient is given a return appointment for the in-office DOT treatment.

The DOT or TUMT therapy takes about forty-five minutes. The heat is applied through a small, flexible catheter that is inserted into the penis. There is no cutting or incision at all, though there is minimal discomfort. This special catheter delivers the exact amount of heat needed to destroy the obstructive prostate tissue. The treatment usually results in the long-lasting relief of all symptoms of

BPH. In my clinical experience, no men have had problems with erection or ejaculation as a result of the DOT or TUMT treatment.

As with any medical treatment, the microwave therapy is not for everyone. One thing is for certain: microwave therapy has dramatically advanced the nonsurgical agenda in the treatment of benign prostate enlargement.

Call the Roto-Rooter Man

In some cases, the large size of the prostate or the severe degree of bladder outlet obstruction requires a more aggressive approach. Nowadays, with the advent of incredible medical technology, prostate operations for benign disease do not even require a surgical incision but can be done through the penis.

This method of treating prostatic obstruction is the transurethral prostatectomy (TURP), a technique that uses either laser ablation (GreenLight laser) or electrocauterization. Almost all benign prostatic obstruction can be cured in this manner. Some of my patients have dubbed this the Roto-Rooter technique.

As with the standard cystoscope, the TURP or GreenLight laser involves entering the prostate through the urinary channel. The ingenious laser beam, or cutting and coagulating device, is inserted, enabling the doctor to core out the obstruction (the compressed hole in the doughnut). This method is quick, relatively painless, and is by far the simplest and safest nonincisive surgical method of relieving prostate obstruction.

In most cases, patients do not need to be hospitalized at all. They usually return home within twenty-four hours, and the recovery period is painless and brief. Unlike the old procedure, which required an abdominal incision, there is little chance of postoperative penis weakness. As one of my patients so eloquently told me, the procedure resulted with him "pissing like a racehorse."

If, like Jerry, you are a superpotent man and you were capable of getting firm erections *before* a TURP (done with or without a laser), you will be just as potent after the procedure. It may be that your penis power is enhanced. This may happen not because of what the surgery does to your genitals, but because reversing the effects of prostate enlargement—distended bladder, abdominal bloating, pelvic pain, and rectal pressure—can improve your general well-being, and with it your sexuality.

If you suffer from an enlarged prostate and your physician determines that all conservative treatment options have been exhausted, do not hesitate to correct a prostate problem with these routine transurethral procedures due to fear of losing your penis power. Your fear is unjustified. The prostate is a secondary sex organ. It is not directly responsible for erection or ejaculation. If you are scheduled for prostatic surgery, you can look forward to sitting through a movie and sleeping through the night without having to run to the bathroom. You will free your mind of anxiety by knowing that your penis will continue to bring you the pleasures you had before.

There is, however, one possible side effect of a TURP (with *or* without laser ablation) that must be mentioned: retrograde ejaculation. In about 30 percent of post-TURP patients, little or no semen comes out of the penis during ejaculation. Instead, when the patient climaxes, semen is ejaculated *backward* into the bladder.

This may sound alarming. Retrograde ejaculation is harmless. The ejaculate is actually evacuated with the next passage of urine. Naturally, retrograde ejaculation presents an obstacle to fertility. The condition is more disturbing psychologically than medically. It does not affect the sensation of orgasm.

A few of my patients have told me that backward ejaculation "makes sex about 10 percent less fun." I cannot personally vouch for that estimate, but I suspect that the minor reduction in enjoyment is because men feel strange about this new process. Most men get used to it and even laugh about the fact that their partners find sex far less messy than it was in the old days.

Regardless, retrograde ejaculation is a small annoyance to accept for the sake of curing benign prostate enlargement and urinary obstruction.

Prostate Cancer

Other diseases that afflict the genitourinary system carry with them a much greater threat, both to life and to penis power. I refer principally to cancer.

Prostate cancer is one of the most serious health problems in the global community. It has touched almost every family by involving either a member or a friend. It is the most common male malignancy. Prostate cancer is the second most common cause of death from all neoplasms (tumors).

Recently, the rate of prostate cancer among men caught up to that of lung cancer. More than two hundred thousand cases are detected each year in the United States alone. About one in every six men in the United States will develop the disease during his lifetime. The rate of incidence increases dramatically with age. Sixty percent of those afflicted are over the age of sixty-five.[1]

In the last thirty years, there has been a dramatic increase in the number of cases of prostate cancer detected each year. This is due to the rising median age of our population, as well as our ability to detect the tumor at an earlier and more curable stage. With the PSA (prostatic specific antigen) blood-screening test, transrectal prostate ultrasonography, and heightened public awareness, the increase in the number of cases is being met with an increase in effective treatment. When patients learn they have prostate cancer, they often assume that they will end up permanently impotent. "You might as well cut off my penis!" they lament. In almost all cases, their fear is totally unwarranted.

Treatment depends on a number of factors, including the patient's physical condition and the type and stage of the cancer cells at the time of diagnosis. In many cases, the recommended treatment is a total nerve-sparing prostatectomy. This entails surgically removing the *entire* prostate gland as opposed to removing only the portion that obstructs urine flow (as is done for benign prostate disease). This is done by creating only a coin-sized incision. A laparoscope (a fiberoptic microcamera instrument) and the da Vinci robot, a revolutionary computerized surgical device, assist in the procedure by providing incredible magnification and enhanced dexterity to the surgical hand. With the advent of the da Vinci technology, the surgical approach to treating prostate cancer has taken a giant leap forward.

As far as sex is concerned, the prostate is a secondary organ. Your penis can perform perfectly well without it. In the past, the old surgical cure for prostate cancer left 60 to 80 percent of patients impotent. The surgery damaged the vital nerve bundles that make erection possible. Today, urologic surgeons utilize a more precise nerve-sparing procedure that has dramatically reduced the incidence of postoperative penis weakness. Approximately 80 percent of our patients emerge from their recuperation with their full penis power intact. The other 20 percent get help with the aid of Viagra, Cialis, Levitra, injection therapy (Prostaglandin E-1), or occasionally a penile prosthesis.

The most essential aspect of ensuring the preservation of normal life expectancy and a high quality of life is the early diagnosis and prompt treatment of the prostate cancer. If prostate cancer is detected while still confined to the prostate gland itself, the cancer can *almost always* be cured with the preferred laparoscopic da Vinci robotic nerve-sparing surgical procedure.

The approach to treatment varies and is heavily dependent on the extent of the prostate cancer at the time of diagnosis. The prognosis is best in organ-confined disease (meaning a cancer that has not yet spread to other parts of the body). Utilizing the laparoscope with the da Vinci robot avoids severing any muscle tissue. This is the key reason this surgical procedure has had especially good results with regard to restoring continence (urine control) and maintaining erectile function. Based on the improved understanding of the anatomy of the neurovascular bundle and the continence mechanism, the newest surgical techniques have made this surgery safe and effective.

Despite the new and improved techniques, surgery is suitable only for those patients whose cancer is completely confined to the prostate gland without any evidence of extension beyond the capsule (outer shell) of the prostate or into the adjacent lymph nodes.

The key to early diagnosis and potential cure is a yearly digital rectal examination by a qualified examiner, a PSA blood test, and an ultrasonic-guided prostate biopsy, if needed. Once the diagnosis of prostate cancer is made, the key to treatment is based upon the underlying stage of the disease. It is essential to differentiate between prostate cancer that is entirely confined to the prostate gland and prostate cancer that has spread beyond the margins of the gland.

The development of magnetic resonance imaging (MRI) has revolutionized prostatic imaging and the staging of the disease. For the first time, we can visualize the internal architecture of the prostate gland prior to surgery. With this sophisticated and precise ability to observe the position and extent of a tumor, we can map all of the tissue around the prostate; we can view neurovascular bundles, seminal vesicles, venous complexes, and regional lymph nodes.

In properly selected patients, surgery can provide a disease-free survival rate of up to thirty years, comparable to the expected survival rate of similarly aged healthy men. To determine which patients are candidates for surgery, the disease's natural history (that is, its biological aggressiveness) needs to be weighed against the patient's life expectancy. Life expectancy is based on risk factors referred to as comorbidities. These comorbidities are heart disease, hypertension, diabetes, obesity, and family history.

As a general rule, if a patient has organ-confined prostate cancer and, in my judgment, his life expectancy is ten years or greater based on actuarial statistics, the patient is an excellent candidate to have his cancer surgically removed utilizing the laparoscopic robotic technique. He can then look forward to living a full and rich life, never again to be plagued by the thought of prostate cancer shortening his life.

My first obligation as a urologic surgeon is to do the best cancer operation I can for the patient. If the prostate tumor has extended to the adjacent nerve bundle, then I will cut the nerve bundle to remove the malignant tissue. Most patients would agree that a surgeon's primary responsibility is to effectively obliterate the cancer. Preserving the patient's life sometimes requires a sacrifice of penis power. Surgeons do everything possible to avoid that contingency, but when it is absolutely necessary, we make the choice knowing that we can take further steps later to help restore penis power.

Since most cancers, particularly those diagnosed at an early stage in older men, are slow-growing, there has been some controversy about treatment. There is published data that examines "watchful waiting" as a legitimate treatment option.

It is essential that the patient be sufficiently informed about the available modalities of treatment so that he can express his preferences about treatment options. There must be shared decision making between a knowledgeable physician and the patient.

The other modalities of treatment that should be considered when the patient is deemed curable include pinpoint IMRT (intensity-modulated radiation therapy) and the implantation of radioactive seeds, or a combination of both. Though modern radiation therapy and the "seeds" have been very effective, it is important to recognize that the disease-free survival rate of patients treated with the radiation option is not as good as for those treated with surgery if the tumor is confined to the prostate.

A number of other treatment options have been publicized. These include cryotherapy (freezing) and thermal therapy (cooking). As of this writing, there is no reliable long-term data available to assess their true effectiveness in eradicating the disease.

Up to this point, we have restricted our discussion of prostate cancer to the more favorable scenario—a cancer that is confined to the prostate alone. With more advanced prostate cancers, including cancers that have spread beyond the confines of the prostate gland, there is still a lot of hope for fully curing the disease. Even though patients in this category are not candidates for surgical removal of the tumor, well-established treatment with hormonal manipulation, radiation, and chemotherapy (often in combination) offers excellent results.

Patients must educate themselves as much as possible. Patient awareness not only makes my job easier, but it also allows the patient to assume a proactive and participatory role in the treatment process. Published data has shown that screening using the PSA blood test in conjunction with a standard, digital rectal examination doubles the detection rate of early prostate cancer.

There is no way to actually *prevent* prostate cancer—not by diet or activity, nor even by picking one's parents wisely. We must turn to early diagnosis to beat the deadly potential of this disease. If you are unfortunate enough to be a victim of prostate cancer, you can survive, live to an old age, and in the end, die of something else.

I have had thousands of patients in my clinical practice who lived long and productive lives with prostate cancer, many of whom did not die of prostate cancer. With a thorough examination, the ability to make a timely diagnosis is nearly 100 percent. If the diagnosis is made early enough to allow the maximum effective treatment, life after prostate cancer surgery or other treatment can be rich and rewarding. It will allow a man to be continent, sexually active, and vigorous in all areas of his life.

A similar situation exists for other cancers in the genitourinary tract. Remarkable new technology enables us to diagnose cancer of the bladder and kidneys at an early stage. This technology allows us to treat those conditions in ways that preserve penis power. Even where the surgeon is forced to remove the bladder, prostate, vas deferens, and seminal vesicles all at once, the patient can still get an erection as long as that vital bundle of nerves is spared.

Testicular Cancer: The Lance Armstrong Theory

Testicular cancer, which affects mainly younger men, is relatively rare. This form of cancer is the most easily treated of all tumors in the genitourinary system. Just twenty-five years ago, more than 90 percent of patients with certain types of testicular cancer did not survive five years. Now, a majority of cases are curable.

Consider the incredible story of champion athlete Lance Armstrong. After being diagnosed with testicular cancer that became metastatic (spread) to his brain, he underwent the removal of the cancerous testicle. He underwent extensive chemotherapy and radiation therapy and came out completely cured. After this trying medical experience, Lance went on to set multiple world records by winning the Tour de France, a race that is arguably one of the most rigorous and demanding of any sporting event in the world. He did this seven times!

His victories are not only a testament to his own incredible willpower but also to the result of a successful cancer treatment. Without the amazing advancements of modern medicine, none of it would have been possible.

In most cases where surgery is required for testicular cancer, we remove one of the two testes. Cancer rarely affects both at the same time. The surviving gonad will compensate by producing additional testosterone. Even if we have to remove both testes, we can preserve normal masculine functioning with testosterone injections, patches, or topical gels. These treatments maintain normal levels of circulating serum testosterone.

Kidney Transplants

Kidney failure is another serious condition that deserves discussion. The main reasons for kidney failure include uncontrolled diabetes, cardiovascular diseases such as hypertension or arteriosclerosis, chronic kidney infections, and viral diseases. For some patients who undergo kidney transplants, the penis power prognosis is not so good. Most patients who require kidney transplants have one or more of these severe underlying disorders, many of which have a negative effect on erectile function and libido.

While most of my patients with only *one* kidney transplant often maintain penis power, those forced to undergo a second transplant typically report erection failure afterward. This happens because the blood supply that ordinarily serves the penis is "borrowed" for the newly transplanted kidney. Many patients with kidney failure are on dialysis while they wait for an organ suitable for transplantation. During that phase, I have noted that libido and sexual function usually decline. In addition, more than half of my patients on chronic dialysis develop penis weakness based on the effects of their underlying disease, certain endocrine complications, and psychological despair.

When a good matching kidney is found and the transplant is successful, a patient can expect to return to a healthy sex life with an abundance of penis power. This is especially true for those patients who have a good handle on their underlying disease. For those men who suffer from diabetes, hypertension, or other cardiovascular disorders, the best thing you can do is to assure meticulous supervision of your illness and do everything in your power to improve your health by seeking medical help and following the advice of your doctors.

The Good News

Now that we have examined the physical conditions that can diminish or destroy penis power, I must emphasize a few important points. The disorders we have discussed in this chapter are not a death sentence to penis power. Only *some* diabetics, *some* men with nerve disease, *some* hypertensives, and *some* cancer patients become impotent. The conditions we discussed might produce only a *partial* loss of penis power, or even none at all.

In many cases, the impact on penis power can be reversed with medical treatment or lifestyle changes. This can be done by giving up destructive substances, by controlling diabetes with diet and insulin, or by improving blood flow with better nutrition, appropriate medication, and exercise.

Even with bona fide organic disorders, a significant portion of penis weakness is psychological. Men who suffer from organic diseases are already saddened by the diagnosis of their illness. They are usually physically weak and emotionally vulnerable. When these patients learn that such organic disorders can cause erection problems, the thought alone weakens penis power in all but the most self-confident and positive men.

As with any setback, attitude is vital. A sick man with a positive mind-set will find ways to continue enjoying his sexuality to the maximum extent possible. I have found that a man with a superpotent attitude can retain his penis power regardless of his physical condition, even if he has to stretch his imagination and alter his sex habits. He can do this completely, even if he has to drastically limit his activities.

I have had patients confined to wheelchairs who adapt to their circumstances and forge a new, superpotent way of life for themselves. Ultimately, where there is penis power, there is a way.

Chapter 6

Blue Pills and Other Medical Cures for Erectile Dysfunction

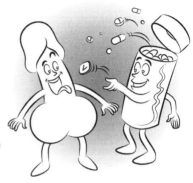

Even for men with true physical loss of penis power, there is hope. Modern technology has enabled medical professionals to help men with superpotent attitudes to function as normally as possible, even those with irreversible organic impotence. The progress in this area has been so remarkable that about three-quarters of what we now do could not have been done even five years ago. Let's look at some of our options.

Blue Magic: The Saga of "the Pills" for Men

No single development over the past thirty years has changed the landscape of men's health as dramatically as the recent widespread use of erectile dysfunction medication. Urologists refer to these medications as "the pills."

Prior to 1997, the only options for the treatment of impotence involved "body-shop" mechanics. These methods included the surgical implantation of a penile prosthesis (similar to a breast implant) and the use of a vacuum erectile device (VED). This particular device, which has the look of a toy, is often seen advertised in the back of men's magazines. The last days of the twentieth century heralded the arrival of the "magic blue pill." Viagra, by Pfizer, revolutionized the treatment of erectile dysfunction.

The drug, known as a PDE-5 inhibitor, was discovered serendipitously. It was first developed as a vasodilator in the treatment of hypertension and coronary artery disease. But after the initial clinical studies were completed, it became apparent the drug was not very effective for this purpose. The manufacturer asked for the male patients involved in the study to return the drug. However, to the manufacturer's surprise, few did.

When asked why they refused to return the unused samples after the drug study was closed, the patients replied that after taking the drug, they obtained the kind of firm erections they remembered only from their youth.

That was the beginning of the revolution. Currently, three erectile dysfunction drugs are on the market, all of which have a similar chemical structure. Viagra was the first to be introduced commercially. This was followed by Cialis, a similar drug whose effects last longer. Cialis was followed by Levitra, which has a profile similar to that of Viagra. All three of these drugs operate in the same way.

To obtain a proper erection, the pills must be taken thirty to sixty minutes before sexual activity. The penis still must be stimulated, either physically or psychologically. If a patient takes any one of these drugs and expects an erection to occur magically by looking at the ceiling, the outcome will be disappointing (unless, of course, there is a picture of a swimsuit model on the ceiling!).

The mechanism of action is the same for all three of these drugs. The main chemical at work is a PDE-5 inhibitor. This chemical boosts the enzyme that relaxes the smooth muscle cells inside the penis. Sexual excitement combined with the drug enables the arteries in the penis to widen and the spaces in the erectile chambers to fill with blood. As the veins in the penis expand, they trap blood in the penis for a prolonged period of time. In tests of all three drugs, men with varying degrees of impotence benefited from the pills in 60 to 80 percent of the trials. These drugs seem to be remarkably effective in patients who have an organic (biological) reason for their impotence. However, these drugs seem to have very little impact on men who are getting adequate erections, but who hope to make sex better (i.e., men who use them as "performance-enhancing" drugs).

It's Not Candy

It is important that men and women understand that these pills are not aphrodisiacs. They are not sexual cure-alls. They will not work in the absence of desire, nor will they make an erection any harder than normal or make it last any longer. Remember that almost all aspects of sexuality (attraction, desire, arousal, and orgasm) remain 99 percent between the ears. When the brain is stimulated by sexual fantasies or by touch, it sends a signal through the nervous system directly to the penis. The signal releases a substance in the penis. This substance is nitric oxide (commonly known as laughing gas and historically used by dentists for anesthesia). The release of nitric oxide causes the relaxation of the smooth muscles within the penis and allows blood to flow freely into the spongy tissue of the penis. This produces a firm erection.

At the same time, the veins that take blood out of the penis constrict. This constriction prevents the blood from flowing out of the penis, keeping it trapped in the spongy tissue until the sex act is completed. These pills inhibit the chemical that breaks down nitric oxide. It is this breakdown process that causes one to lose an erection. By blocking the breakdown of nitric oxide, these drugs create a longer period of smooth muscle relaxation in the penis. This mechanism allows the penis to stay erect for a longer period of time.

These pills are not "desire" drugs. They are "capacity" drugs. They do not create desire; more accurately, these medications give a man the *capacity* to exercise his sexual potential.

Lovemaking, and sex in general, is much more than an erect penis simply interacting with someone else's body for the sole purpose of releasing sexual tension. The sexual experience must go far beyond its physical characteristics. It must involve intimacy, sensuality, and an emotional connection based on respect and caring. Couples with problems in their interpersonal relationship should not turn to these drugs as a quick-fix solution. These drugs are designed to help individuals revive and maintain the sexual aspects of a healthy, intimate relationship. They should not be used as a substitute for resolving conflicts. Communication and discussion are more valuable than any medicine.

If you and your partner have extenuating issues in your relationship, an active sex life might create the illusion that everything is all right. Ultimately, the underlying reasons behind a conflict must be resolved before a complete and healthy relationship can exist both inside and outside the bedroom. The hard fact is that these "magic pills" cannot accomplish this goal.

Use with Caution

A partner with erectile dysfunction is often angry, depressed, and frustrated. This is especially true if the couple has not had sex in a long time. For this reason, if the pill is effective, major psychological and physical adjustments must be made in the sexual perspectives and practices of both partners. The fact that each of these pills takes about thirty minutes to work is the good news. This allows time for intimacy, tenderness, and foreplay.

On the other hand, if a man takes the pill without informing his partner, gets a firm erection in about thirty minutes, and then assaults his partner without preparing her for an intimate experience, he will be viewed as an unattractive aggressor. His actions are certain to weaken the relationship. An impotent man newly empowered by the effects of the powerful pill must somehow communicate tenderness, affection, and intimacy if he hopes to have an ongoing and meaningful sexual relationship with his partner.

A man cannot sneak up behind his mate at any random time and say, "Hey, look at me, I have a firm erection—bend over and let's make love!" That kind of behavior not only has the potential to offend your partner, it also ultimately works against the process of developing and maintaining a meaningful sexual relationship.

The key to the best use of these drugs is *communication*.

Prior to the introduction of the pills, it was my clinical observation that the men who suffered from erectile dysfunction would usually shy away from any verbal or physical expression of sexual desire. They feared raising false hopes in their partners. Their partners, in turn, also avoided sex out of fear of inducing guilt in their counterparts. They may already have been plagued by penis weakness and the anxiety of not being able to have a firm enough erection for penetration.

If a couple wants their sexual interaction to be anything more than physical, both partners need to make significant psychological and emotional adjustments in the way they view their sex lives. I have witnessed couples who had significant problems within their interpersonal relationship. Many did not address any of these deeper issues prior to swallowing the pill. In all of these cases, any benefits generated by the ability to "perform" with a firm penis failed to deal with the emotional aspects of intercourse.

My advice to all of my patients is, in fact, to *be patient*. If you are considering taking one of these powerful pills, please take the time to discuss the ways in which this medication will change the nature of your relationship. Resolve underlying frustrations and grievances so that the bedroom does not become a space of denial and escape from the realities of a frustrated relationship. If you are anxious and imprudent and choose to rush through any discussion of the deeper implications of a renewed sex life, this failure to communicate could result in conflicts that seriously strain your relationship. Through patience, openness, and mutual understanding, both partners can ultimately receive the wonderful benefits these pills have to offer.

You Are Not Alone

According to the National Institutes of Health (NIH), approximately fifteen to thirty million men in this country, half of whom are under the age of sixty-five, suffer from some form of erectile dysfunction.[1] It affects about one in four men ages fifty to fifty-four and one in two men over the age of sixty.[2] Data compiled shows that Viagra is effective in about 85 percent of all patients with pure psychological impotence.[3] It is effective in slightly more than 70 percent of men whose inadequate erections have an organic cause, including neurological disorders, poor blood supply (caused by vascular diseases), or diabetes—or are a consequence of prostatic surgery.[4]

These medications are most effective in patients whose erectile dysfunction has resulted from spinal injuries or from surgery for prostate cancer. The enormous appeal of the pills is their ease of use. They can be taken orally and discreetly. They can be taken many hours prior to the desired time for erection. Unlike the injectable medications (e.g., prostaglandin-E, Caverject), which produce an erection regardless of stimulation, the individual *must* be sexually stimulated in order for any of these pills to work.

These drugs are prescription medications and should not be taken without a thorough evaluation by a competent urologist or other qualified physician. Impotence is often an early indicator of a potentially serious underlying vascular or endocrine disease. There-fore, taking any of these drugs without a full medical evaluation could complicate many of these conditions to a life-threatening de-gree. If a patient with erectile dysfunction has silent, undiagnosed coronary heart disease and he takes any of these drugs, he could suffer a fatal heart attack while having intercourse.

Though all of these pills are relatively safe and carry minimal side effects, they are still very potent drugs. Even though they can cure a significant life-*altering* condition (i.e., erectile dysfunction), the underlying cause of the dysfunction can be a life-*threatening* condition. These drugs should never be used in patients who are taking any form of nitrates, such as nitroglycerin, organic nitrates, or "poppers" (amyl nitrates). These drugs are all chemicals com-monly used in patients with coronary artery disease. The most sig-nificant side effects of the pills are minor and include headaches, facial flushing, nonspecific back pain, alteration in perception of the color blue, and heartburn. In my practice, the most interesting fact is that very few men discontinue use of the pills due to these side effects.

When a patient comes to me in distress about penis failure, the first thing I do is reassure him that everything will be all right. Once we define the cause of the dysfunction, we can assign an ap-propriate treatment option. With the pills, we start with the lowest prescribable dose (Viagra 25 mg, Cialis 10 mg, and Levitra 10 mg) and slowly move up to the maximum prescribable dose if needed.

If the oral medications are not suitable or they are not work-ing for you, other corrective treatments might be more beneficial. These treatments include injection therapy, an intra-urethral sup-pository (Muse), hormonal therapy, or in some cases a surgical prosthesis.

There is no doubt that these pills have worked *magic* for millions of men currently suffering from impotence. But their use must be approached with caution and with the understanding that they may not help all men with impotence.

Remember, all of these drugs have the ability to dilate blood vessels. When these drugs are taken in combination with certain other drugs, particularly nitroglycerin, there may be a sudden drop in blood pressure. Sometimes this may lead to death. It is very wise before using any other drugs to check with your doctor to see if there is any possibility that a drug in your medicine cabinet may interact with the PDE-5 inhibitors. The pills have inherent potential health dangers. Their indiscriminate use can mask serious underlying medical conditions. Please heed my advice: see a doctor before taking any of these drugs!

Do Not Let the Hype Fool You

The long-term effects of continuous and large doses of any of these three pills (Viagra, Cialis, Levitra), especially when men are taking them for marginal reasons, remain unknown. In the end, these pills are a long way from the magic potion the media hype would have us believe them to be, particularly in men with significant underlying medical conditions or advanced age.

Speaking of the media, I have come to find that male and female magazines, movies, and television shows often create an ideal of perfect sexuality. People watching these shows believe they have to live up to certain standards of sexual behavior that are dictated by the media's portrayal of the inner motives of women *and* men.

These standards are in most cases completely unrealistic. Within this idealized realm, anything less than being a perfect, Herculean lover is unacceptable. In my clinical experience, most women *do not* want their partners erect for twelve hours. The advertised phrase— "If your erection lasts longer than four hours, call your doctor" (Cialis)—seems, at first glance, like the primal rally cry for all superpotent men. In fact, most women are more than satisfied with ten to fifteen minutes of intercourse surrounded by tenderness and expressions of intimacy. When asked, most women outright reject an "erection marathon."

When I observe the use of the pills within the homosexual community, I find that gay and bisexual men are four times more likely to use the drugs for marginal or recreational reasons. These individuals are also more inclined to view a long-standing erection as a badge of honor. Unfortunately, use of the pills in the gay community is often associated with the abuse of narcotics. This is especially true at sex parties. These parties often include not only the use of crystal methamphetamine but also the use of drugs such as cocaine, ecstasy, or ketamine. The combination of these drugs with the pills can and does result in serious cardiac or neurological problems, or both. There is also an associated spread of sexually transmitted diseases, including HIV and AIDS.

Men taking medication for HIV infections are not only more likely to suffer from erectile dysfunction but are also much more *sensitive* to the effects of the oral medication. Certain protease inhibitors, the mainstay of treatment for HIV-positive patients, can markedly increase the blood concentration of Viagra, Cialis, or Levitra. This may result in the magnification of both the effectiveness of these drugs and their potential side effects. Therefore, in HIV patients taking these drugs, the smallest possible dose of the PDE-5 inhibitors must be used to achieve adequate performance levels and safety margins that are acceptable.

From Pills to Pellets: The Muse System

There is another relatively new drug that is commonly employed to correct erectile dysfunction. It utilizes a very effective chemical known as alprostadil, or prostaglandin-E (PGE-1). In the past, this active chemical was only available for direct injection into the penis using either the Caverject or Edex system.

Many of my patients find the thought of injecting a tiny needle into the base of the penis unpleasant, painful, inconvenient, and in many cases impossible to master. Luckily, there is a more advanced delivery system that uses a drug marketed as *Muse*. This system also uses alprostadil (PGE-1), but employs it with a new and unique application system. The system is an intra-urethral suppository.

With the new Muse system, the drug is delivered by very carefully inserting a small, soft pellet into the tip of the penis, where it comes in contact with the urethral mucosa (urinary channel). The pellet dissolves almost immediately. The drug is promptly absorbed into the bloodstream, causing rapid dilation of the vessels in the penis. This results in a firm erection. There are minimal side effects, which might include minor urinary discomfort.

Muse is the only noninjectable delivery system for this powerful drug, PGE-1. It should only be used in men who have had a failed response to the oral therapy (i.e., Viagra, Cialis, Levitra). The Muse system usually produces an erection within five to ten minutes after application. Based on what we know so far, it is both safe and effective. Using Muse is quite simple. I ask the patient to urinate first, then insert the applicator one inch into the tip of the penis. The patient then gently pushes a button on the top of the plastic applicator and an effective dose of Muse (the urethral suppository pellet) is delivered to the urethral membrane. We usually start with the lowest dose of Muse (125 or 250 mcg) and increase the dose as necessary. At the present time, I am recommending a maximum frequency of use of no more than one system per twenty-four-hour period.

Muse appears to provide consistent effectiveness regardless of the underlying cause of erectile dysfunction: diabetes, blood vessel disease, neurological disorder, postsurgery side effects, trauma, or psychological problems. The most serious local side effect so far has been priapism. This is the medical term for a persistent and painful erection. The risk of this appears to be less than one-half of one percent. I must emphasize the need for a physician to calculate the proper dosage of Muse. The most commonly reported side effect is mild penile discomfort, particularly associated with urination. Overall, the Muse system is well tolerated and is an effective alternative to the oral therapy.

As with all of the drugs used for erectile dysfunction, my patients are delighted with their improved emotional well-being and the enhanced quality of their interpersonal relationships. These improvements are attributed to the restoration of satisfactory intercourse. Unlike Viagra, Cialis, or Levitra, with the use of the Muse system, erections occur automatically. This means there is no need for sexual stimulation. In the properly selected patient, the Muse system is an excellent alternative for the treatment of erectile dysfunction.

Shooting It Up: Injectable Medication

When the normal circulatory events that result in a good, firm erection cannot take place due to a physical disorder, urologists can produce instead a perfectly functional *pharmacological* erection. Our preferred method is to inject a medication into the shaft of the penis. The main drug used is prostaglandin-E1 or PGE (the same chemical used in the Muse system). PGE is a vasoactive drug that relaxes the smooth muscles in the walls of the penile arteries. It also increases blood flow into the corpora within the penile shaft through vessels that are commonly blocked by arteriosclerotic plaque. The results are dramatic! The penis becomes semierect within five to ten minutes. It becomes quite rigid in fifteen minutes. In most instances, it remains erect for thirty to fifty minutes. Significantly, the drugs have no effect on orgasm or ejaculation.

The safe use of the injectable medication began nearly three decades ago. We are still confident in the effectiveness of this treatment method. With the use of this technique, we have restored thousands of penis-weakened men to active, fulfilling sex lives. After assigning the proper drug and then determining the precise dosage for each individual patient, we meticulously train the patient to inject himself. The system uses a tiny needle and a small syringe similar to those used by diabetics who self-inject insulin.

Once we are satisfied that the patient has mastered the technique, we instruct him to inject the medication prior to intercourse. It is simple and painless. The results are automatic. The injection will produce an erection even in an anesthetized patient. Interestingly, however, the effect can be modified by external stimuli. Erotic stimulation *enhances* the effect of the medication. This occurs because stimulation increases the presence of the circulating neurotransmitters released by the brain when it is sexually aroused. These chemicals complement the dynamics of the drugs. By contrast, we have seen that the lack of privacy in the doctor's office can *reduce* the effect of the drugs. So the good news is that the drugs tend to work better in the bedroom than in the examining room.

These drugs must not be used without strict medical supervision. Our instructions must be followed precisely, and active follow-up is essential. Because of possible side effects, certain men should not use injectable drugs. These are men with conditions such as varicose veins, a condition in which blood tends to pool in the limbs, men with blood disorders such as sickle-cell anemia, and men with unstable cardiovascular disease and symptoms such as fainting spells. Those who have limited dexterity or poor eyesight—both of which could lead to errors when preparing the syringe or injecting the medication—should also avoid using these injectable drugs. Additionally, I am very cautious about prescribing this method for patients who I consider emotionally unstable. As with any drug, there is potential for misuse. In such cases, I strongly recommend psychological counseling before I administer the drugs.

One possible misuse of injectable drugs is to take them too often. I am reminded of one patient in particular, an extremely wealthy man in his sixties who had had a history of superpotent activity. He reacted with anger when a vascular condition rendered him physically impotent. He had just married a much younger, world-class beauty. I prescribed a "vasoactive cocktail." This was a combination of PGE-1 and papaverine. I determined the proper dosage, taught him how to self-inject, and off he went to his home in Europe to spend time with his new wife on their yacht in the Mediterranean.

From time to time, he called to let me know that everything was great. When he returned to Los Angeles, he came in for a checkup and raved about the therapy. He said he was having the best sex he'd had in thirty-five years—three times a day, sometimes for hours at a time. He could not have been happier, and I could not have been more alarmed.

I had specifically instructed him to inject the medicine no more than once every other day. I told him that what he was doing was dangerous. "How can it be dangerous?" he replied. "You always told me that sex is great exercise. I feel fabulous!"

That was not the point. I was concerned with the potential side effects of medically inducing erections six hours a day! The danger is *priapism*. If an erection lasts too long, the blood trapped in the penis does not drain. This can result in permanent damage to the delicate sinusoids within the penis and may lead to impotence so severe that not even injectable drugs can counteract it.

Priapism is the most serious complication that can result from this form of therapy. It occurs very rarely, almost always after the misuse of medication. When it does occur, we have to act quickly to avoid permanent damage. We instruct patients to phone us or the paramedics immediately if an erection lasts longer than four hours. If that should occur, the patient is instructed to come in immediately. We inject a Neo-Synephrine solution directly into the shaft of the penis to gradually reduce tumescence (erection). In many cases, we often give patients an emergency syringe with a proper dose of neo-synephrine to be kept at home.

Other side effects that sometimes arise from injection therapy include dizziness, headaches, a metallic taste in the mouth, bruising or inflammation of the penis, tingling sensations, and swelling or angulation after the injection. Most of these local complications are minor. They can be avoided if the patient follows our instructions to the letter.

Those instructions are extremely rigorous. The use of self-administered injections is one of those areas where "informed consent" is vital. My staff and I spend a great deal of time with the patient and his partner explaining the action of the drugs, the theory behind the therapy, the proper dosage and application, and the risks and possible side effects. Each patient is also given a packet of printed material to take home with him for further information.

One of the main considerations for the urologist is to determine the appropriate *combination* of drugs to be injected and their proper dosages. Not all men react the same way to a given dose of a vasoactive drug. We have to find the precise amount and create a custom-designed "recipe" for each patient. The ideal combination is exactly what is needed for that patient to achieve the goal—an erection that lasts thirty to forty-five minutes without side effects. The ideal dose varies depending on the underlying cause of the problem, the patient's state of mind, and the psychological environment in which he takes the drug.

Only after meticulously testing various doses in my office under controlled clinical conditions do I teach the patient to self-inject. We never allow a patient to administer drugs on his own until we are certain that he has mastered all the necessary skills.

Patient response to the treatment varies. At one extreme are patients like the newly married, wealthy European man who are so satisfied with the effects of the treatment that they abuse the privilege. At the other extreme are those individuals who discontinue therapy either because they are afraid of possible complications, squeamish about injecting themselves, or turned off by the loss of spontaneity caused by having to stop and inject a drug into their penis. The majority of patients fall in the middle.

This majority is made up of those who are grateful for the medical technology that enables them to have a satisfying sex life. They are grateful to achieve superpotency despite their medical limitations.

Surgical Procedures

I am often asked if I can transplant penises the way I can kidneys. The answer is an emphatic no.

At this point in time, we are unable to electively transplant an appendage such as the penis. The penis has unique functions depending on a complex mix of nerve, blood, and hormonal variables, all hinging on delicate feedback mechanisms. With all my faith in modern science, I cannot imagine a time when impotent men will be rejuvenated by the surgical transplantation of real genitals. Even if the technology existed, we have so many simpler alternatives that I doubt it would ever be used.

Since many erection problems are caused by insufficient blood flow to the penis, medical science has naturally sought methods to reverse that problem. Studies so far have focused on ways to transfer blood from neighboring vessels to the deep arteries of the penis. These surgeries, which are still largely ineffective, have demonstrated some success in young men suffering from acute pelvic trauma. However, due to the complex vascular anatomy of the penis, we have been unable to duplicate the success we have had with coronary bypass surgery and the treatment of other arterial disorders.

Experimental work has also been done on the other side of the erection coin—preventing venous leaks. An erection cannot be maintained unless the veins in the corpora hold in the blood. With modern diagnostic procedures, we can tell when blood is leaving the venous channels in abnormal amounts. Although work in this area is still in its infancy, surgery can be performed on selected patients to impede the backflow of blood from the penis and reverse the effect of a venous leak.

Pump It Up: Implants

The most common *surgical* procedure for impotence is the implantation of a penile prosthesis. The combination of ingenious design, technical proficiency, and durability has made it possible for us to implant prosthetics *directly* into the penis. In recent years, a variety of devices have been developed that enable surgeons to easily implant this device in an outpatient hospital setting. This has provided urologists with a permanent solution for thousands of organically impotent men who have a commitment to penis power and the motivation to undergo surgery.

The implants allow for complete sexual satisfaction with a very low rate of failure. At one point in the late 1980s, about thirty thousand prostheses were implanted each year around the world. Since the introduction of the injectable medication (PGE-1), and more recently with the arrival of oral therapy (Viagra, Cialis, and Levitra), the number of prostheses has declined. This decline has not been as dramatic as one would think. This is largely due to increased promotion in the media for treatment of erectile dysfunction and the resultant creation of a larger pool of prospective surgical candidates.

There are basically two types of prostheses. The older variety is the so-called malleable implant, which consists of semirigid rods that are placed into the corpora (the sausage casing–like bodies that normally fill with blood to create the erection). These implants make the penis rigid enough to successfully penetrate. The problem with these types of devices is that they do not change in length or girth. This means that the man has to walk around with a semifirm penis at all times. The device is flexible enough to bend into somewhat of a concealable shape, but the penis looks a bit unnatural. It may be a source of some embarrassment at the health club!

The second type of implant is the inflatable prosthesis. This consists of two inflatable cylinders that are surgically implanted in the same corporal channels. It also includes a pump and a fluid-filled reservoir, usually implanted either within the scrotum or lower abdomen.

When the patient desires an erection, he simply squeezes the pump several times. The fluid flows from the reservoir into the cylinders. The cylinders expand and swell, mimicking a natural erection. After intercourse, a release valve is simply pressed. The fluid flows back into the reservoir, returning the cylinders to their empty state. The penis returns to its flaccid state. It is quite an ingenious design.

Because the inflatable model allows the user full control and leaves the penis looking relatively normal, this type of implant is much preferred by my patients. However, it requires a slightly more extensive surgical procedure. This implant has a higher rate of malfunction than the malleable type, which has no moving parts or fluid connectors. Correcting mechanical failures is not like opening the hood of your car and replacing a spark plug. These surgical corrections require another surgical incision.

When I first began to implant the inflatable devices about fifteen years ago, they were frequently plagued by mechanical failures. These failures often required repeat surgeries. Recent improvements by manufacturers (particularly AMS) have been dramatic. The technology on the horizon promises to be even better.

I predict that if inflatable prostheses continue to be profitable for manufacturers, the research and development dollars will be allocated. This will lead to nonbreakable components that produce erections indistinguishable from the real thing.

A word about *my* mind-set. Before considering a patient for a prosthesis, I meticulously rule out all *correctable* medical conditions. For me, implantation is the treatment of last resort. When the decision is made, I inform the patient of the pros and cons of all the available devices. I still recommend the malleable device for many obese patients. If the penis is partially hidden by a protruding belly, its artificial firm appearance is not usually noticeable.

With a slender man, however, the semirigid device stands out like the proverbial sore thumb. Once the choice is made, the device is implanted, usually under regional anesthesia. One cylinder is placed in each corpora cavernosa ("sausage casing"). The surgical incision is small. It is buried unnoticeably in the scrotum. The procedure takes about thirty to forty-five minutes. Complications during and after surgery are extremely rare. Postoperative discomfort is relatively short-lived. The body tolerates the implant almost as if it were made of flesh and blood.

Each prosthetic is customized for the individual patient. The device has to be tailored to fit the precise length and width of his corpora. We cannot implant a prosthesis that is smaller or the erections will have a floppy tip—the so-called SST deformity. This deformity is named after the droopy nose of the Concorde supersonic transport plane. We also cannot implant a device that will make the penis longer, despite the fantasies of many patients. In other words, after prosthesis, the functional penis, both erect and flaccid, will be the exact size it was before the implant.

For the Right Reasons

The ideal candidate for a prosthetic implant is someone with all of the mental characteristics of a superpotent man, but one who is unable to achieve a satisfactory erection because of a real medical disorder. I remember a patient of mine who was from a distant country, a country with a vastly different culture from our own. One of the wealthiest men in the world, he had been married for thirty-five years to a woman he loved. He also had a concubine, an accepted custom in his society. This man had fathered approximately one child a year for nearly twenty years. He then developed diabetes. This became so severe that he was unable to have normal intercourse. After considering all the alternatives, he opted for a penile prosthesis. Ever since the surgery, he and his loving wife (and his concubine as well) have been grateful that the penis power that never left his heart was restored to the rest of his body.

For the Wrong Reasons

Thinking of that man's renewal brings to mind another gentleman from that same part of the world. This gentleman represents the perfect example of the *wrong* reason to have a prosthesis. A member of a royal family, he came to my office at age forty-two for a urologic problem unrelated to sexuality. When I examined him, I noted that his penis looked quite misshapen and that he had a primitive prosthetic device. This device had been implanted when he was only twenty-seven! Years ago, the available devices were crude, even in America, and his device had been implanted in a Third World country. This country was not at the cutting edge of medical technology. Visually, the result was grotesque.

He asked me if I could improve the appearance of his penis. Surgically, I could not. However, I was curious as to *why* he chose to have the operation in the first place. He had no organic illness, yet before he was even thirty, he had chosen to endure the pain, embarrassment, and risk of having a crude plastic device implanted in his penis.

His reasons were as repulsive as the prosthesis itself. He was enormously wealthy and could afford to buy and have anything in the world. He owned all the homes, boats, planes, cars, and toys that a man could possibly dream of. At the snap of his fingers, he could have an entourage of beautiful and willing women—and he snapped his fingers routinely, particularly when traveling outside his strict, conservative nation. He had everything money could buy; however, he could not buy the number and frequency of his erections. They were limited by physiology. So he *bought* himself an unlimited erection.

This was not a superpotent man. His warped view of the penis and its power represents the best possible reason for *not* having a penile prosthesis.

A more typical candidate whom I routinely discourage from having an implant is the eighty-year-old retired man who comes to me for a routine prostate exam and offers the news that he "cannot get it up anymore." He wants a prosthetic like the one a friend of his has. The surgery has restored his friend's sex life, so why not his? Upon questioning, the following scenario is typically revealed: he has been married to the same woman for more than forty years, and the marriage has brought him more aggravation than joy. He is in reasonably good health but is often a sour, bitter man with very few interests and low self-esteem. He has, in effect, given up on life. There is nothing wrong with his sexual apparatus that a change in attitude and a renewed zest for life or a change of habit would not cure. In such cases, I advise *against* the implant.

You might ask why I said no to him when I had performed the operation on his friend. The reason is that the friend was a man in his late seventies who had stayed involved in his business and enjoyed a variety of recreational activities. He was a spirited man and a widower who was involved with many younger girlfriends. Ultimately, he was a good candidate because he was a superpotent man. His penis power was not up to his penis demands. This was due to a vascular problem that had necessitated bypass surgery. This man was a perfect candidate for an implant; his grumpy friend was not.

Mechanical Devices

For impotent men who seek an alternative to surgery or self-injection, there are several other devices on the market. The most popular of these fall under the heading of "external vacuum therapy." Vacuum erectile devices (VED) produce erections by mimicking the physiology of oral sex. They use *suction*. First, a plastic cylinder is placed over the penis. A vacuum is then created with a pump. This draws blood into the penis, causing it to expand. When the penis becomes rigid enough for penetration—usually in a minute or two—the patient removes the cylinder and places a rubber band–like constricting device around the base of his penis. The band impedes venous outflow so that the erection can be maintained long enough for successful intercourse.

Vacuum erectile devices manufactured by reputable companies are safe. The advantages of VEDs are low cost and minimal risk of side effects. VEDs preclude the need for surgery, medication, or injections. The disadvantages of VEDs are that they are awkward to handle and take a few minutes to assemble. This reduces the pleasure and spontaneity of lovemaking. Rarely, the ring or rubber band used to impede the outflow of blood can inhibit ejaculation.

Vacuum therapy is a reasonable alternative for many men, especially those who suffer from *partial* loss of erection or fear prosthetic implant surgery or injecting themselves with drugs.

Professionally and personally, I would highly recommend good old-fashioned oral sex! It has the same effect as a VED. In fact, it is even better then a VED because it is performed with the loving warmth of your partner's body and not by an inanimate object.

Mechanical devices should be used under the supervision of a physician. Patients with blood disorders like sickle-cell disease or clotting problems should not use these devices. Healthy men able to get satisfactory erections should not use a VED as a performance enhancement device. It is dangerous, and such abuse would be the antithesis of penis power.

Aphrodisiacs and Other Substances

Nearly every culture in every period of history has a record of substances alleged to stimulate sexual desire and improve virility. These have been derived mostly from plants. They range from the infamous Spanish fly to complex combinations of Chinese herbs.

Others include L-arginine, Gingko, ashwagandha or "Indian gin-seng," the Mexican herb damiana, and the plant extract called pygeum. Sadly, nearly an entire species of magnificent white rhinos have been slaughtered just to macerate their horns in the fruitless pursuit of penis power. Medical science has found no evidence that these aphrodisiacs work. Perhaps they have a placebo effect. I have found no ingestible animal part or herbal substance that will cure penis weakness.

There is one herbal substance that may have some merits. It is *yohimbine*. Derived from the bark of the yohimbine tree, it has been considered an aphrodisiac by native cultures for hundreds of years. Initial studies have substantiated the claim. Dr. Christiaan Barnard, the eminent heart surgeon who pioneered human heart transplantation, used yohimbine on patients who developed im-potence after surgery. He reported satisfactory results in 75 per-cent of his cases. However, mainstream medicine does not embrace yohimbine therapy. Yohimbine's biochemical action is not under-stood. The original research was contaminated because yohimbine was used in combination with other drugs, primarily testosterone. So far, there is little reason for me to think that the bark of a tree can foster significant improvement in men with penis weakness.

Beware of possible dangerous side effects if alternative treat-ments are used. One of my patients, in a dicey self-experiment, applied a nitroglycerin paste to the shaft of his penis. Because of its "vasoactive" profile, he concluded that it could increase penile blood flow. He eventually had to stop using it. During sex, the sub-stance was absorbed by his wife's vaginal mucosa, giving her severe headaches. The same might be true of the off-label use of minoxidil, which is marketed as an aid to hair growth in balding men. Because it also is a vasoactive substance, some have suggested that rubbing it on the penis might produce better erections (or even hair!). I urge you to refrain from self-experiments with such products. There are plenty of proven alternatives.

Men all over the world spend billions of dollars every year in search of a magic elixir that can potentially cure penis weakness. For every man out there in need of a cure for penis weakness, there are dozens of hucksters hawking snake oils and cure-alls that have no verifiable scientific merit. As a physician, there would be no reason for me to withhold legitimate, effective therapy for erectile dysfunction from my patients. It is important for the public to understand that a scientific process exists for proving the effectiveness of any therapy, which consists of a double-blind, controlled, crossover study that justifies its use. I recommend to all my patients that they refrain from using any drug or substance that does not meet the strict standards of scientific inquiry.

In summary, men who have a superpotent mind-set but are limited by illness or injury can reclaim their penis power with medical help. The medical advancements in the area of erectile dysfunction have been magnificent, and I would predict even further developments in the near future. However, only a small percentage of men with penis problems have true organic impotence. The vast majority of men have normal, perfectly capable penises served by well-functioning auxiliary organs. There is nothing physically wrong with these men and their penises. For millions of men, surgery, drugs, and mechanical aids have no place in their lives. The answer for them lies between their ears.

Chapter 7

Performance Anxiety: When It's All in Your Head

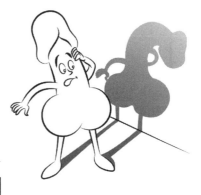

S omething's wrong with me, Doc," said Steve, a thirty-nine-year-old lawyer. "I want a complete urologic workup."

I asked him what the trouble was. "I met this great woman," he said. "We had a terrific time on our first date. She invited me in, one thing led to another, and before I knew it we were in bed. But I . . . well . . . I couldn't . . . you know . . ."

I knew all right. I had heard it so many times before from hysterical patients. Steve was terrified that something had gone wrong with his penis, when in reality his failure to get an erection with his terrific new woman had nothing to do with physiology. He had gone through a bitter divorce. It had taken him some time to get used to being single again. On the ill-fated date, it was the first time in many years that he had even kissed a woman in earnest other than his wife. Steve was not impotent, he was just plain nervous. The newness of the experience, the excitement of meeting someone he liked, and his eagerness to please her and prove himself a worthy

123

bed partner all conspired to create one of the greatest enemies of penis power: *anxiety*, or more precisely, *performance anxiety*.

More penis weakness occurs the *first time* a man is with a particular partner than at any other time. When it happens, men feel so humiliated that they sometimes find any excuse they can to avoid dating that person again, thereby depriving themselves of what might have been a good relationship. It is sad. I have even met men who, after several embarrassments, stayed away entirely from people who turned them on. They became, in effect, celibate prisoners of penis performance anxiety.

It happens a lot with younger men. Take, for example, a college freshman named Cliff. He was plagued by premature ejaculation and erection failure. In high school, already uncertain of his masculinity and misled by the bravado of his buddies, Cliff's earliest sexual experiences were disasters. He kept trying, and because he was a handsome, rugged young man, he had no trouble finding dates. When the sex did not work out, he was so mortified that he never tried it with the same girl twice. His *first* times got even worse because his performance anxiety increased with every bad memory. Eventually, he stopped dating altogether, except to perhaps escort a date to a safe social event. In college, he created a fictitious out-of-town girlfriend. In fact, Cliff was as horny as a devil and tired of masturbating. He finally got up the nerve to tell me about his "mechanical problem."

His sexual self-esteem had taken such a pounding over the years that he was finally convinced that he needed medical help. After I examined him, we sat down in my office. "You do not have a mechanical problem, Cliff," I told him. "You have an attitude problem." I assured him that his early sexual experiences were not unusual. It is like getting back on a bicycle after you fall: you just have to do it. In his case, preferably with the same bicycle. I encouraged him to find a girl he liked and stay with her long enough to feel calm and trusting when they were in bed. I added, "If things do not go right the first time, do not panic. If the girl has a heart, she will under-stand, and the next time you will be much more relaxed."

Cliff was relieved to hear he was not sick. Within a short time, he fell in love with a sweet, understanding girl and embarked on a steady, sexually satisfying relationship.

The first time with a new sexual partner can be an exciting ex-perience. For some men, however, that very emotional excitement can lead to temporary penis weakness. It can spiral into a pattern of disaster. It happens to many young people like Cliff. It can happen to grown men who have been out of circulation like Steve. In cases like Steve's, the same advice applies: take your time, be patient, stop pressuring yourself, and stop thinking you are inadequate. Find a partner who makes you feel comfortable and unthreatened. It worked for Steve, and it will work for you. You must be willing to face the challenge with the courage it takes to overcome perfor-mance anxiety.

If you find yourself overwhelmed in a sexual encounter and your temporary penis weakness leads to impotence, there are medical solutions for you. As an emergency measure, you can always carry a few Viagra, Cialis, or Levitra pills, but only as a last resort and after consulting with a urologist to be certain it is safe for you to use any of these strong prescription drugs. (See chapter 6, "Blue Pills and Other Medical Cures for Erectile Dysfunction," for more on "the pill.")

If you do choose to turn to the pills as a solution, beware of the "crutch effect." The crutch effect can occur when you use a pill once and it works. You then conclude that you will never get an adequate erection without the drugs. Becoming dependent on drugs as a solu-tion to penis weakness does not address the real problem. Until you are willing to find the confidence to face your fears about sex and intimate relationships, you will never overcome penis weakness.

Anxiety Is Penis Power's Archenemy

The stories in this chapter will help you understand that first encounters can be just as traumatic as they are exciting. There are a lot of reasons for temporary penis weakness. They may have nothing to do with physical problems.

Let us start with an in-depth examination of *performance anxiety*. In my practice, it is the leading cause of penis failure. Performance anxiety is much more likely to happen when you are with an unfamiliar partner or when you feel pressured to measure up to some hypothetical sexual standard.

What you perceive to be a *physical* problem is more likely in your mind. The cause is usually something simple and obvious. Performance anxiety can be fixed with a change of perspective or a change of circumstances. It is important that a single disappointment not make you believe that you are less of a man or that something is wrong with your penis. Losing an erection once in a while is as much a part of sex as booting a ground ball is to a shortstop or missing a target is to a marksman. If and when it happens, you have to be able to move on. If you hold on to the memory of the failure, it will surely become the seed of future disappointments.

Accentuate the Positive

Take a lesson from successful men in other fields. When I meet men in leadership positions, I observe that they never think in terms of failure. They do not even use the term. They prefer "mistake" or "error" because the *f*-word implies a certain finality or permanency that they are not willing to accept.

Successful people focus on positive goals. Successful people put all their energy into the task at hand. They do not look back, they do not make excuses, and they are not intimidated by setbacks. If things do not go well, successful people analyze the situation and use the lessons they learn to carve out future triumphs.

Of course, you have to learn the *right* lessons from your setbacks. That was precisely the problem with Cliff and Steve. They drew the *wrong* conclusions. The idea they came away with was "There must be something wrong with me." That is not the attitude of a successful man in any field, and it is not the attitude that will fortify your penis power.

Management expert Warren Bennis coined a term that captures the superpotent attitude as it relates to performance anxiety: the *Wallenda Factor*. He named it after the world-famous aerialist Karl Wallenda, also known as the "Flying Wallenda." When Wallenda stepped out on the tightrope with nothing but air between him and the ground, he *never* thought of failure. He was fearless, seemingly impervious to the danger of falling. He did not even think of *not* falling or *not* embarrassing himself. His full attention was on what he had to do at the moment. For fifty years, Wallenda was known as the most fearless and flawless aerial acrobat. Unfortunately, while Wallenda's career illustrates the importance of having the right attitude, his ultimate fate demonstrates what can happen if you do not have the right attitude.

In 1978, before walking a tightrope seventy-five feet above the ground, Wallenda was different for some inexplicable reason. According to his wife, "All Karl thought about for three straight months prior to it was *falling*. It was the first time he'd ever thought about that, and it seemed to me that he put all his energy into *not falling*, not into walking the tight-rope."[1] For the first time in his career, he personally supervised the installation of the rope and checked to see that the guide wires were secure. It is believed that because of his preoccupation with falling, the great Wallenda fell to his death.

Metaphorically, this is exactly what Cliff and Steve and millions of other men do when they approach sex with their minds consumed by the fear of failure: they end up defining their goal as "not embarrassing myself" rather than "having a good time." Having any kind of negative perspective is going to prevent both you and your partner from extracting the maximum pleasure possible from a sexual encounter. Take a lesson from Wallenda: do not think about failing, do not think about past setbacks, and do not think about anything other than the task at hand. Direct your attention completely on the sensual experience of making love.

Even the Strong Are Let Down Sometimes

What can be done if you do have performance anxiety? Let us start with the issue of anticipating the use of your penis. When you begin to feel anxious or fearful, you are programming your mind for failure. Stop what you are doing, calm yourself down, and remind yourself of what Winston Churchill, with cigar in mouth, so elegantly and succinctly stated during the World War II London blitz: "There is nothing to fear but fear itself." Losing an erection, unlike carpet bombing, is not life-threatening. What is the worst thing that could happen? You embarrass yourself? You can only be embarrassed if you let yourself be. If you think that a "real man" cannot possibly lose an erection or ejaculate too quickly, then you will be encouraged to know that these things happen to *every* man at some point in his sexual life. So why should you be embarrassed if it happens to you? And what if you *are* embarrassed? How bad is that really? Maintaining this positive point of view will keep you calm and lighthearted. If you feel that way, your penis is likely to behave accordingly. If you develop the ability to laugh at both yourself and that unpredictable appendage of yours, you will both be winners.

Get rid of fearful, negative thoughts altogether. There is no valid reason to entertain them. They are the natural enemy of your penis. Mobilize a battalion of positive thoughts, and let them take over your mind. *Penis power is the power of positive thinking applied to your penis.*

I have had patients report back to me and say, "Well, Doc, I did what you said, and I was *still* nervous." Sometimes the fear is so deep-rooted that you cannot bring yourself to believe in your own pep talk. As you fill your brain with positive thoughts, another part of your brain is snidely whispering, "Bullshit!" My advice is to keep those positive thoughts coming. Work at it relentlessly. In the long run, even the most cynical disbeliever will be convinced. With perseverance, your conviction will manifest into a positive penis attitude and ultimately will result in reliable penis behavior.

It is a fact that some men with a deeply rooted fear of penis failure need more than just a pep talk. Perhaps a prescription for Viagra, Cialis, or Levitra is just what is needed to break the vicious cycle. However, the "crutch effect" may result in dependence on these medications. I often suggest that patients talk to a psychotherapist and perhaps explore deeper reasons for their anxieties. In most cases, lack of self-esteem is the underlying cause. Their self-image is so low that it affects every aspect of their lives, not just sex.

Unfortunately, it is much easier to compensate for low self-esteem in business or sports than it is in bed. Surprisingly, many men who are plagued by self-doubt are successful professionally. But *your penis never lies and your penis is never fooled*. Your penis is a perfect reflection of your deepest thoughts and emotions. If you *think* that you have no self-esteem problem and that you are a pretty terrific guy, but you worry about your sexual performance, then you may harbor some doubts about your masculinity. Self-doubt travels from the brain to the penis in a flash.

You might have to work on your basic self-esteem, either with the help of a counselor or on your own. Basic questions to ask in evaluating your level of self-doubt include the following:

• Do you constantly compare yourself to other men?

- When something minor goes wrong, do you scold yourself or call yourself insulting names?
- Do you judge yourself more harshly than you judge others?
- Do you find yourself trying hard to please other people?
- Do you strive to be liked by everyone?
- Are you overly sensitive to the criticism of others?
- When you do something well, do you belittle your accomplishment?
- Do you have a strong need to prove yourself?
- When faced with a new challenge, do you immediately worry that you will not measure up?

If you answered yes to most of those questions, then self-doubt is part of the problem. If that is the case, your penis will pick up on your lack of self-acceptance. If *you* do not think you are capable of good, solid penis performance, then why should your penis act otherwise? If *you* do not think you deserve a fully satisfying sex life, then why should your penis give you one?

Everything possible should be done to raise your self-esteem. Look at all the positive things you have accomplished. Try to look at all the kind, generous things you do. Look at all your admirable traits. Examine the standards by which you measure yourself. Self-doubt comes from the failure to live up to what you expect of yourself. If what you expect of yourself is based on standards that are imposed by other people, social institutions, or the media, then you are not being true to yourself. Who says that you are supposed to live up to some arbitrary standard? Who is to say that you are less of a man if you do not look or dress a certain way, or that you have to be with a certain type of person, have sex in certain positions, or sleep with some predetermined number of people? What's most important is to recognize who you are and what your values are. Do everything you can to live up to those personal standards and goals. *Set your own penis standards and then evaluate yourself with a fair and generous perspective.*

After making these changes in your self-image, your self-esteem will improve. If you are still having trouble expressing your penis power, there are alternative solutions. As we discussed in chapter 6, the erectile dysfunction drugs Viagra, Cialis, and Levitra can help you *temporarily* overcome performance anxiety. Remember well, though, that when penis failure is not due to an organic problem, the use of these drugs is only a provisional solution. It is undesirable for any man to depend on chemicals to help him achieve what is naturally possible. At the same time, to help men overcome the initial anxiety caused by penis failure, and as an aid in building performance confidence, the pills are an acceptable "bridge" mechanism.

Lighten Up, Dude

Okay, you are in bed with a sexy partner, whether it is your wife of thirty years or someone you just met. You feel tense. You start to worry that your penis will not get hard or that you might lose the erection that just popped up. What do you do? Your first reaction might be to panic. You might worry so much about your penis that tension builds. You get clumsy. You try to exert your willpower on your organ. You forget about doing all the things that might excite your partner. You cannot appreciate, or even feel, the kisses and strokes your partner is so lovingly giving you. One of two things is bound to happen next: your partner gets turned off and thinks he is doing something wrong or your penis goes limp. From my experience, it is usually both.

The minute you start to feel any anxiety, stop what you are doing immediately and *tell* your partner about it. Do not make excuses. Do not try to hide it. Own up to it. Explain openly that you are nervous, that this sometimes happens to you. It happens to all men. Tell your partner you want so much to please her, bring her satisfaction, and that her acceptance means a lot to you. Make sure she understands that it is not her fault, she is terrific, and she has not done anything wrong. Tell her it is all in *your* head, and it will surely go away.

Honesty is always the best policy in general, but when it comes to your penis, it should be the *only* policy. Ninety-nine percent of the time, candor will improve the situation by diffusing tension. If you have a healthy relationship, your partner will understand. Your partner will appreciate your integrity and your vulnerability. Most people want intimacy, affection, and closeness in bed, so if you communicate these qualities, your partner will not hold your anxiety against you. He will probably reassure you, calm you down, and take the pressure off. If your partner does *not* act this way, or if he gets angry, gets resentful, or demeans you in a castrating way, you should ask yourself if you are in bed with the right person.

And if you *do* fail to get an erection? If you *do* lose it at precisely the wrong moment? If you *do* ejaculate too quickly? What then? I say laugh it off! You are probably thinking, sure, that is easy for the doctor to say. But I mean just that. Joke about it. Lighten up! I assure you that "real men" can and do laugh at their own penises. They might say funny phrases to their partners like "Oh well, that rascal pulled a fast one on me," "I cannot get him to behave sometimes, the unpredictable little devil," or "Do not take it personally." Remarks like that, expressed in your own words and your own style, should ease the tension and help your penis rise another day, or even the same day. Medically, I can practically guarantee it.

Your partner should appreciate the light touch and will be pleased to know that you are trying to improve your sexual ability. She might start thinking that something is wrong with *her*. She might be feeling guilty for failing you. She might know you feel ashamed but not quite know what to say or do about it. You can take the lead and break the ice with a good laugh. Who says sex has to be serious?

When you get right down to it, with all the unstated agendas, the physical clumsiness, and the childlike awkwardness, sex is just as suited for slapstick comedy as fine art or soft-focus cinematography. Many people say there is no better turnon than a good, hearty laugh in bed, and nothing sexier than a partner whose sense of humor is compatible with your own. Just do not take your penis so seriously. That is how the trouble starts in the first place.

If you do not succeed, try again and again and again. Do not shy away from using your penis if it falls down on the job once or twice—or any number of times. Do not give up on it. Practice makes perfect in sex, just as it does elsewhere in life. Perseverance is the only way to get over setbacks and gain the confidence you need to overcome your fear of failure. As a last resort, you can always turn to your urologist for the quick but temporary fix provided by medication.

In discussing issues of self-confidence, I am reminded of a former patient of mine whom I'll call Joe. Joe was a short man with a classic Napoleon complex. He had gone from one business to another, becoming fabulously successful in each one before moving on to the next challenge. A bachelor at forty, he talked so much about the women he dated that I assumed he was having a healthy, varied sex life. To my astonishment, this human dynamo was plagued by penis weakness. It stemmed from an absence of self-esteem. All of his accomplishments, it turned out, were a workaholic's futile attempts to gain the approval he never got from his father. His father was a domineering man who raised his son to be emotionally fearful. Joe lacked self-confidence. Joe saw himself as worthless. When he was alone with a woman, he perspired from fear, not passion, and most of the time, his performance was the equivalent of bankruptcy.

Joe had one great attribute: perseverance. In everything he did, he was a determined, "never say it's over" kind of guy. When he finally recognized and admitted to his dissatisfaction with his penis performance, he delivered the same determination to the bedroom that he delivered to his work. A therapist helped him deal with his self-esteem, and I evaluated him urologically. I assured him that he was fully capable of attaining penis power. Very soon after this boost in confidence and morale, his sexual relationships blossomed.

Joe offers a stark contrast with another patient whom I will call Daniel. Daniel also suffered from crippling self-doubt and penis weakness, only he expressed it in the opposite way from Joe. He was a classic *underachiever* in all aspects of his life, including sex. An outstanding guitarist, he had been a child prodigy and excellent student. His low self-esteem kept him from realizing his potential. It prevented him from capitalizing on his appealing looks and likable, self-effacing personality. At twenty-nine, he eked out a living teaching guitar. He spent every night alone. Daniel had not had a date in over a year. A series of disappointing experiences relegated sex and romance to pure fantasy. Daniel lacked what Joe had: perseverance and the courage to expose himself to possible failure in order to conquer his fear. Daniel is still wrestling with self-doubt and trying to generate the courage to try again. He is like a child too scared to get back on his bicycle after taking a spill.

Perseverance is usually essential to succeed at most things worthwhile. Whenever I think of perseverance, I think of a certain country lawyer who lost his job, lost an election for the state legislature, failed in private business, failed to land a nomination for Congress, and was twice defeated for the Senate. He did all of this while persevering enough to earn some victories and ended up one of our most revered presidents. So the next time you are ready to give up on your penis, think of Abraham Lincoln.

There is a caveat to that advice: *persevere, but do not try too hard*. If you try *too* hard, you might make things worse. Joe, my Napoleonic patient, was one of those guys who approached every task with a full frontal assault. That is how he bolstered his penis power. Becoming superpotent is not like making a better business deal or improving your tennis game. Some tasks succeed because of hard work and effort. Getting an erection is not one of them—the more you work at it, the less likely you are to succeed. It is analogous to falling asleep. Anyone who has ever tossed and turned with insomnia can tell you that the harder you *try* to sleep, the more agitated you become and the longer you stay awake.

It is what I call the "Penis Paradox": *the harder you try, the softer it gets*. You cannot will your penis to get hard or stay hard; you cannot implore it, order it, command it, or force it. The anxiety of trying to get an erection works against the natural process of getting one. As with sleep, you just have to create the right conditions and stay out of the way. Initially, Joe had *more* problems when he decided to conquer his penis weakness. He tried *so* hard to perform well that he could not relax enough to get an erection. Only when he learned to calm down, let go, and simply enjoy what he was doing did nature take its course. From that point forward, his perseverance began to pay hefty dividends.

Your penis *wants* to get hard. That is what it does. That is its nature, just as your heart wants to beat, your lungs want to breathe, and your stomach wants to digest. They are all involuntary functions. Getting an erection is no different. Believe in your penis. Trust it. Give it every opportunity to do its job, but also give it the freedom you would give a trusted friend or colleague. Allow it to pursue its mission without you meddling or worrying. Just stay out of its way!

Don't Worry, Be Superpotent

Anxiety in any shape or form is the worst enemy of your penis, and I do not just mean anxiety about your performance. If you are nervous about finances, the health of a loved one, your child's college application, some business situation, or some other troublesome aspect of adult life, your penis might let you down, even if you have great faith in it. Worries and fears are physically debilitating.

Worry and fear cause wear and tear to the endocrine and nervous systems. Worry and fear cause the blood vessels throughout the entire body to constrict. How could they *not* affect your penis?

Do not allow fear to enter your bedroom! Park your anxieties at the threshold. In fact, park them out on the street. Do not let anxiety near where you make love. The trick is to learn how to *compartmentalize your life*. My most well-rounded, superpotent patients come by this skill naturally. Business is business, play is play, family is family, religion is religion, and sex is sex. They do not mix things up in their practice or in their minds. No matter how stressful things are at the office, the minute they leave the building, they leave the stress behind. They never allow it to pollute their family lives, and especially not their sexual performance. If their kids are goofing off at school, if their roof is leaking, or if their in-laws are hounding them—even if their mechanic said fixing the car would cost a small fortune—they leave these domestic hassles outside the bedroom door.

If you find it difficult to compartmentalize, you will have to work at it. If at any time irrelevant, negative thoughts intrude on your penis performance, start by mentally pushing those thoughts aside. Consciously send them away and shift your attention to the erotic sensations you are experiencing as you make love. For some people, shifting attention is as easy as switching channels on a television. Others need to work at it the same way they have to work at changing any old habit—and negative thinking is often just that—a *habit*. A psychologist colleague of mine recommends a visualization exercise that can help you clear anxiety from your thoughts.

In your mind's eye, see yourself gathering up your troubles and placing them in a box. Then watch yourself seal the box and put it outside a door or toss it out of a window. It may sound ridiculous to people who view their feelings as some sort of forbidden territory. However, if you are willing to try to make changes in your relationship with your body, then these techniques can really help you along the way.

Get those worries out of the bedroom, and give your penis permission to do the thing it likes to do most without interference. Focusing on and entertaining certain emotions like anger or resentment is a very nonproductive way of coping with the troubles we may experience. There are healthy methods for dealing with stressful or troublesome situations. The most important principle is to *not* become enraged or filled with anxiety. It is crucial to acknowledge your emotions. Be honest about what you are feeling. Talking about frustration and anger with someone you trust is good. Unfortunately, too many people allow their emotions to spin out of control. Heed this advice: wild and uncontrolled emotions will only pollute the rest of your life. Accept things for what they are, do what you can to make them better, and move on. These are essential steps in becoming confident in your penis performance. Emotional balance is a basic element in becoming a superpotent man.

In the pursuit of the pleasures of penis power, I suggest cultivating what British philosopher and scholar Bertrand Russell called "the habit of thinking of things at the right time." The bedroom is not the place for planning next week's schedule, rehearsing a speech in your mind, or worrying about tomorrow's board meeting—especially if you are concerned about something over which you have no control. Russell wrote, "The wise man thinks about his troubles only when there is some purpose in doing so; at other times, he thinks about other things or, if it is night, about nothing at all."[2] Russell was referring to sleep, but if you want to be a superpotent man, apply the same thoughtlessness to penis activities as well.

One way to help keep anxious, worrisome feelings from inhibiting your penis power is to burn off some of your stress with exercise. Volumes have been written about neutralizing the effects of stress with physical activity. There is no need to take up space here with the rationale for this advice. However, it might make it easier to compartmentalize before you get intimate with your lover if you lift some weights, run a few miles, swim a few laps, play racquetball, take a yoga class, pound a punching bag, or walk on the beach. Take advantage of any modality to burn off stress and relax your mind before you get into bed.

Better yet, burn it off *in* bed. That is right: the best way I know of to get rid of stress is to have sex. Here we have another Penis Paradox:

> Stress can interfere with penis power, but at the same time, exercising your penis power is a terrific way to eliminate stress.

I cannot count the number of superpotent men who have told me that their favorite antidote for their high-pressured professional lives is to hurry home to their partners. Sex is a great physical exercise, and it is a great way to release tension. It is wonderful for clearing the mind, and it has fringe benefits that other activities cannot approach: sharing affection, experiencing intimacy, and feeling good about yourself. It bests almost all ills. If you can learn to channel your frustration, anger, and worries into sexual energy, you can turn the tables on stress. That is what great performers do. Instead of letting anxiety debilitate them, they use it as an energizer and a motivator. Great performers channel it into their performances, and that real emotional energy is what can make a performance spectacular. Do not let anxiety diminish your penis power; use your penis power to diminish your anxiety.

I once said exactly that to a Hollywood talent agent whose workday was like a nightmare cooked up by the phone company and the makers of ulcer medication combined: one high-pressure phone call after another. It was destroying his penis power. He did not have the ability to compartmentalize. "Do not wait until after supper and the kids have gone to sleep and you are passing out on your feet," I told him. "Grab your wife and go to bed when you get home and burn off that stress before it burns you."

A week later he told me he could not do it. Why? Because he felt guilty. He thought his wife would feel he was abusing her and having sex with her only to satisfy his own physical needs and not because he wanted to share the joy of lovemaking with her.

This was a noble thought from a man who truly loved his wife. It was also irrational. He was having penis problems as a consequence of all that stress. Knowing his wife, I urged him to follow my advice in spite of his reservations. My hunch proved to be correct. His wife thought hopping into bed for a quick, aggressive workout was romantic. She was only too happy to help her husband burn off the stress. The result was he did not carry the stress with him all night.

If you have a good, loving relationship, your partner will not feel exploited if you use sex to combat stress. He would prefer to see you calm and collected rather than nervous and worried. If you take care of his needs at the same time you are satisfying your own, you will both end up winners.

Depression Depresses the Penis

Another of the many patients who have come to me thinking they were penis failures was a sweet, gentle man named Bill. He worked at my hospital as an orderly. A divorced father of three, Bill suddenly developed a bad case of penis weakness after two years of a healthy sex life with his girlfriend. It did not take long to figure out why. Taking a routine medical history, I found out he had also been sleeping badly and losing weight. When asked about his state of mind, Bill replied he had been depressed recently. His son was addicted to cocaine and had been caught stealing to support his habit. In addition to the deep sadness anyone would feel over this misfortune, Bill was plagued by feelings of helplessness and remorse. He felt that he could not help his son.

Nothing was wrong with Bill's sexual apparatus. His penis power had not disappeared. It was on hiatus because of situational depression. Loss of interest in sex is a common and predictable response to deep sadness or personal loss. Situational depression made sex the last thing on Bill's mind. Instead of just accepting his depression and letting time take its course, he made things worse by forcing himself to have sex with his girlfriend. He feared his girlfriend would think less of him if he said he did not feel like making love. He already blamed his son's problems on his own shortcomings as a father. Bill thought it would make him even less of a man if he did not have sex. He went about lovemaking on schedule, but he could not lie to his penis; it was not ready to perform. Bill's sexual energy had gone into a slump, along with his appetite and his zest for life's joys.

Depression is a serious obstacle to superpotency. In Bill's case, it was a temporary condition brought on by an identifiable situation. Once he understood the impact of situational depression, Bill was able to accept the fact that his reaction was normal. In time, he got over the pain, the sadness dissipated, and his good life—including his aroused penis—returned.

In other cases, depression can be a chronic, debilitating disease. Its effect on penis power can be long-lasting. Such conditions are beyond the scope of a urologist. If you have penis weakness because you suffer from chronic depression, it would be a mistake to focus on your sexuality alone. Your penis problem is one of many predictable symptoms. I would urge you to see a psychiatrist, who can diagnose and treat your condition properly. Today, medication, psychotherapy, or a combination of both can effectively manage depression. With ascent from the depths of depression comes a natural restoration of penis power.

Mind Games

Martin was a middle-aged man who had lost his wife a year before he came to see me. She was the love of his life. After an appropriate period of mourning, he began to say yes when friends offered to set him up with dates. Martin's first few dates were with sexually liberated women. Things went very well for Martin, considering that his only sexual experiences outside of marriage had been some furtive encounters with girls when he was a very young man. When he finally met a woman he really cared for, he suddenly lost his penis power. Martin could not understand why he should perform well with women for whom he felt indifference and might never see again but not with someone for whom he truly cared.

Martin was plagued by *guilt*. He had no trouble with the first few women because he knew nothing would come of the relationships. They were there purely for fun and to ward off loneliness. When he met someone he truly wanted to be with and the sex became more intimate and loving, he was overwhelmed by the thought that he was betraying his late wife. To spare himself the guilty feelings, his mind "tricked" his penis into falling down on the job.

Martin's case is another example of how penis power can be undermined by emotions. Guilt is a big one. There are many sources of guilt in our society. Social norms for relationships, principles of obligation and responsibility, and of course, certain standards or expectations of behavior all contribute to the presence of guilt in our world. One of the most significant factors behind guilt is religion. Many of my patients—Christians, Jews, Buddhists, and Muslims—were all perfectly fine sexually within the prescribed context of marriage. When they indulged in behavior that overstepped the boundaries of their religious precepts, many were driven to penis weakness. I came to discover that the real culprit was guilt.

My role is not to question anyone's religious beliefs. Every person must make his own choices as to the morals and ethics by which he conducts his life. However, anyone who chooses to violate his personal tenets should understand the consequences: subconscious shame can have dramatic effects on the penis, including erectile dysfunction, premature ejaculation, and even a permanent psychological aversion to sex. In most cases, men who struggle with strict religious rules, especially regarding sex, need to talk to a clergyman and not a urologist.

Fears

Another obstacle to penis power is *irrational fear*. I am not referring to fear of performance failure or other actual threats, but a bizarre fear of a dire consequence when engaging in intercourse. I remember one thirty-year-old man who would have been a virgin had it not been for one woman who coaxed his semierect penis into her vagina. For this young man, all previous sexual encounters had ended in erection failure or ejaculation before penetration. I referred him to a psychotherapist. This therapist discovered that he was raised by a domineering mother who told him as a young boy that vaginas had teeth! He never engaged in sexual intercourse because he was plagued by nightmares about getting his member "chewed up."

That patient was an extreme case, but many men fear intercourse for reasons they do not quite understand. Many do not even realize they are afraid. They think they want to have sex. They seek it out, but something always goes wrong. They conclude that their penises are abnormal. Whether it is the wrath of God, the spirit of their mothers, or vaginas with teeth, some deep fear renders their penises weak.

A major contributing factor to penis weakness is the fear of disease. I have had many patients whose penises failed them because they feared acquiring some highly unlikely disease like typhoid or they were afraid of having a heart attack during sex. These are bizarre terrors rooted in some deeper fear of sex.

Other worries are *not* irrational. Men have very good reason to be concerned about sexually transmitted diseases, whether they be a viral infection such as herpes, a bacterial infection like syphilis or gonorrhea, chlamydia, or HIV/AIDS. All have been on the increase in recent years. While the others can cause suffering and inhibit your sex life, HIV/AIDS has become the principal pariah of sex in our time because it is both incurable and often deadly. The fear of HIV/AIDS has put a definite crimp in the lives of many of my superpotent patients, as well it should.

The time to worry about sexually transmitted diseases is not at the moment of intercourse. You need a game plan long before you get into bed with someone. In today's world, it is incumbent upon a superpotent man to know a potential sex partner as well as possible before having sex. You must have the patience and courage to ask probing questions. You must ask about your partner's past sexual practices and previous partners. You must make a sound judgment on the truthfulness of your potential partner's answers.

With regard to HIV/AIDS transmission, when you are sexually intimate with any given partner, you are potentially linked to every previous sexual encounter in which your partner has ever indulged. Think of the risk the next time you consider having a one-night stand with a stranger or sleeping with a new partner on a whim. You might have to delay your gratification. You could end up saving your life.

On the other hand, if *you* are the carrier of any kind of sexually transmitted disease, your absolute duty is to be open and honest with your potential partners. It could save their lives. If you take sound medical precautions, engage only in safe sexual practices, and exercise sensible sexual judgment, you can be free of fear when it is time to unleash your penis power.

Chapter 8

Extenuating Circumstances: When Sex Becomes a Chore

Larry was a fifty-one-year-old man who came to me for a prostate examination. I informed him that his prostate was indeed enlarged and would require treatment, possibly even surgery. His response was amazing. He was relieved. I asked him why he was so happy to hear that he had a prostate disorder. "Because I've been having problems getting it up lately, Doc," he confessed. "I thought maybe I'd become impotent, so I'm glad to know it's only a minor prostate problem."

"Larry," I said, "I'm sorry to have to tell you this, but your prostate has nothing to do with it. If you're having problems with your penis, the surgery is not going to change anything." As I explained earlier, the prostate's role is to supply seminal fluid to the ejaculate. It is not related to penis power or penis performance.

Larry was now really depressed. We had a long talk about his medical history and his personal life. Larry had been married to the same woman for nearly thirty years. Thirty years of ups and downs, raising children, and dealing with hassles day in and day out. Thirty years of watching each other sag and wrinkle and of routine, habitual sex. Larry was not impotent. There was nothing wrong with him physically. He was suffering from the *Coolidge Effect*.

Researchers studying animal sexuality originally coined a unique behavioral pattern as the Coolidge Effect. You will easily see the relevance for human beings. If you put a male mouse in a cage with a female mouse in heat, he will quickly mount her. After he ejaculates, he will rest before going at it again. The time he takes to rejuvenate—the refractory period—is predictable. It varies from one species to another, but is consistent among all rats, roosters, rams, rhinos, and humans. After the second ejaculation, the male will rest again, only this time the refractory period is longer. The same is true after the third copulation, the fourth, the fifth, and so on. The animal takes longer and longer to recover until it finally reaches exhaustion.

That much seems obvious. Here is the interesting part. If at any point you remove the female mouse and replace her with a different one, all bets are off. It is back to square one for the male. No matter how many times he has ejaculated, introduce a new female and his refractory period bounces back to nearly what it might have been after one or two copulations. This is the Coolidge Effect.

Why that name? Legend has it that President Calvin Coolidge, the austere conservative they called "Silent Cal," was visiting a farm with his wife. Noticing an unusually large number of chicks and eggs, Mrs. Coolidge remarked that the few roosters in the barnyard must be prodigious studs. The farmer proudly replied that the roosters did their duty dozens of times a day. "You might point that out to Mr. Coolidge," said the First Lady.

Evidently, Silent Cal was not as prudish as his reputation suggests. He asked the farmer if each rooster had to service the same old hen every time. When the farmer told him that the roosters could mate freely with any hen they wanted, the president responded, "You might point that out to Mrs. Coolidge."

No one is quite sure if that story is true but, if not, it *should* be, and it certainly deserves to have an effect named after it.

Let us return to the case of Larry. I have seen Larry's problem in hundreds of men. They think something physical is wrong with them when the problem is really a matter of *circumstances*—not their penises. The situations that cause temporary penis weakness are often so obvious that I am surprised they go unrecognized by the patient. Men are so vulnerable to self-doubt when it comes to penis performance that they immediately assume something is wrong with their anatomy.

One of the most common of these circumstances is what Larry described to me as the inevitable boredom and habituation between long-term partners. It is true—sex can sometimes become routine after a while. The thrill of taking off a partner's clothes is not so thrilling when you have unveiled the same body hundreds of times and it parades before you naked every day of your life (one survey found that 51 percent of men fantasize about someone else during sex, while only 37 percent of women do).[1] If your partner of twenty-plus years says she "wants you," it is not quite as exciting as having the same words whispered into your ear by a shapely stranger. Let us be honest: you do not have to be youth-obsessed or an ageist to be more turned on by a young, tight, lithe body than the familiar one that gravity and time have altered. Nor do you have to be sexist; I would wager that the same holds true for women.

The Hard Dick Syndrome

There is no question that new equals exciting, whether it is a new car, a new song, or a new sex partner. Nothing will revive a man more quickly and more vigorously than a new partner, preferably one who is young, attractive, and receptive. That observation may seem subversive to those who value monogamy and cherish the undeniable spiritual and emotional benefits of lasting love. Nevertheless, when it comes to penis power, I have seen the evidence thousands of times. Men who have difficulty making love to their longtime partners can be dynamos with their mistresses or secret lovers. Men can be troubled by penis problems until they get separated or divorced and suddenly find rejuvenation with a new lover.

I am not suggesting that the French have it right by condoning the tradition of mistresses. It is not my place to endorse any particular lifestyle. However, the reality is that penis weakness is often circumstantial, and the Coolidge Effect defines one of the primary circumstances. A surprisingly large number of men, especially middle-aged men, think they are losing their penis power when the only thing that is happening is a predictable lessening of desire due to a sex life built around monotonous routine.

That being said, I hasten to warn men who assume new is always better that such thinking can be dangerous. I have seen too many men jeopardize, and sometimes forfeit, longstanding relationships of immense value because they followed their penises in pursuit of someone new and young.

In many instances, men merely substitute one set of problems for another. Many men solve their boredom problems *temporarily*, only to realize later that they desperately miss the love and companionship they squandered. Their penises are reborn for a little while, only to retreat again when their new, exciting, and secret lives grow stale. *Beware of the hard dick syndrome!* After a while, it can turn into the Coolidge Effect.

Solutions to the Coolidge Effect can often be found within the confines of a good, monogamous relationship. Those same animal researchers found that the male's vigor can return, even without a new female, if something else is altered. This could be a new scent or a unique appearance of the old, familiar mate (the researchers achieved this by painting the female mouse's coat a new color). The lesson here for humans, both male and female, is that like many activities, sex can settle into a dull routine. Familiarity might not breed contempt, but it certainly breeds boredom and disinterest. The ultimate goal is to break your old and tired habits. Change your routines. Use your imagination. Make love in different places or at different times. Wear different clothing. Daub yourself with unusual scents. Try different positions. Experiment with different types of foreplay.

Whatever it takes to bring a sense of freshness and adventure to your sex life, do it! Do not just give up on yourself by thinking you are over the hill or that you have suddenly become impotent.

Problems that stem from longevity and familiarity might seem to contradict something we talked about in the previous chapter: fear and performance anxiety can cause penis failure during first encounters. You may be asking yourself if I am suggesting that being with an exciting new partner for the first time can cause temporary penis failure the same way that penis failure can be caused by being with the same partner for a long period of time. The answer is yes. This is another Penis Paradox.

Both sets of circumstances can cause the same types of problems for very different reasons. "First time" problems are caused because the situation is *too* exciting. The anticipation of sex, apprehension, and anxiety over your performance are psychological factors that become heightened in a new encounter. It is the heightened experience of these emotional factors that can cause you to lose an erection or ejaculate too quickly, both of which are much more common than you may think.

With a longtime partner, the problem is exactly the opposite. The problem arises not because of anxiety or first-time jitters but rather because of diminished desire. When you have been with someone many times, it simply takes more time and more direct stimulation to get aroused. If you do not take that into consideration and do not add some spice and imagination to the routine, you might find that your penis is going, "Ho hum, I cannot get worked up over this anymore." If you are just going through the motions, your penis might just lie down on the job.

We have two sets of circumstances, one diametrically opposed to the other, both of which can cause temporary penis weakness. The solution to the "first time" anxiety is to cultivate a comfortable, relaxed, familiar relationship. If *that* reaches a critical mass and the problem of monotony sets in, the antidote is to generate excitement with freshness and variety.

The Spice of Life

As a urologist, I cannot emphasize this point enough: do everything in your power to prevent sex from becoming a dull routine. Nothing will bring passion and romance back to a long-term relationship faster than a change in sexual practice or venue.

I remember a fifty-five-year-old patient who was married to a woman he loved for twenty-seven years. He had a bad case of sexual ennui (dissatisfaction resulting from boredom), which led to a brief fling with his dentist's assistant. That made things even worse at home because he was now inhibited by guilt in addition to boredom. "Jack," I said, "take Friday off and get your wife to cancel all of her plans. Rent a cabin in the mountains for a weekend. You have not done anything spontaneous and romantic in years. Do it. Tune out the world. No kids, no phone, no television, just the two of you and a fireplace."

The weekend rejuvenated Jack and his wife, as similar escapes have done for countless couples. In other cases, I have advised patients to take the afternoon off and surprise their wives with flowers and a sunset tryst in a motel. Other couples have done things like pretend they have just met and are having a one-night stand. Or they simply vary their rituals. If you have been initiating sex after you are both washed, undressed, and in bed, try doing it before all of those bedtime rituals. When was the last time you and your partner undressed each other instead of starting out in your pajamas? When was the last time you necked in the living room and carried your partner into the bedroom? Or made love in the kitchen or the shower? Have you tried a different position in the last few years? Have you thought of using props? Browse in any sex shop and you will get countless ideas of how to invigorate your sex life. Above all, use your *imagination* and see what you come up with.

Hopefully, you will not have to go to extremes, like the wife in Woody Allen's *Everything You Always Wanted to Know about Sex But Were Afraid to Ask,* who could only have sex in public places. For the majority of people, simply giving yourself permission to break your own boundaries will elevate your penis power several notches. You might have to do some cajoling to win your partner's support. That could be translated into a surprising delight for both of you.

Some of my patients have to be told that it is okay to have sex at different times of the day. They have to be told that sex is not just a nighttime activity. Why engage in something as important as sex when your body is at its lowest energy level? Perhaps your penis problem is really a fatigue problem. The penis responds to different biorhythms, as do hormonal secretions and energy levels. This is an important aspect of understanding the intricate relationship between the penis and the body. Concrete scientific evidence to validate this observation is sparse at this time, but research in this area is ongoing.

I do not doubt that fatigue affects sexual energy. For this reason, I encourage my patients to pay close attention to the ways in which their bodies, and especially their penises, respond to different emotional and physical conditions. It is fundamentally important that you be aware of your body's rhythm. Your sexual responsiveness will change with stress, fatigue, anxiety, or sickness. Your particular rhythms may be better suited to sex at unusual times of the day. Perhaps certain habits, for example exercise, diet, work schedules, are affecting your sex drive in negative ways. Pay attention to the subtle clues your own body transmits, and you will know where to start making changes. Explore all of your options. Experiment, take risks, and mix things up until you find the right balance for your love life to flourish. What's most important is not to feel burdened by sex. If your sex life is becoming run-of-the-mill and boring, then take the initiative to spice things up. You will not be disappointed by the results of reviving passion and romance in your relationship.

Hard on Demand

Millions of men think that something is wrong with them because they do not get "hard on demand." The persuasive myth in our culture has it that a "real" man will be raring to go any time, day or night. That proposition could not be further from the truth. A wide range of difference exists among men. Men have their own individual preferences and unique biological templates. There is simply no set time or place you are "supposed" to get aroused. No credible scientific book says you have to have sex a certain number of times a day to be a "real man." I cannot count the variations. Some men tell me they feel sexiest in the morning, in the middle of the day, at night, or in the middle of the night. The real problem is that most men are just too inhibited to break their old habits, or they are afraid their partners will think they are crazy or weird for trying something new. Even if your requests may seem odd, you still have the power to prove yourself to your partner through your performance. If you are passionate and exciting, your partner most likely will not complain.

Morning sex is an especially good way to break the routine. What a terrific way to start the day! So what if you have to skip jogging, rush through breakfast, or get to work a bit late? Morning sex can be just as invigorating as a morning jog and just as relaxing as a cool morning breeze. It is the best wake-up call. It clears the spirit of any tension and shakes the cobwebs out of your body. In fact, a lot of men like sex better in the morning because they wake up with the so-called "morning wood" or "piss hard-on." The explanation for this morning erection is that a full bladder compresses the venous outflow from the pelvic vessels, holding blood in the penis longer than usual. The usual result is a morning erection. Be assured that after morning lovemaking, you will like what you see in the mirror. You will have set the right tone for a great day.

If you are a man who wants to enhance your penis power, or if you are a partner who wants to learn how to increase your man's penis power, then it behooves you to look into alternative sex practices. Countless volumes have been written on this subject, from the *Kama Sutra* to articles in *Cosmopolitan*. I will not try to reiterate information that's already available. However, ask yourself these questions: When was the last time you tried something other than the missionary position? Have you tried letting your partner get on top and control the action? Have you tried "doggy style"? How about not having intercourse at all, but bringing yourselves to climax strictly with oral sex or mutual masturbation? The possibilities are endless. If you cannot conjure up some creative ideas on your own, do not be afraid to go out and find a book or ask a friend for some good tips. Any change should add a fresh dimension to your routine. I can guarantee that both you and your partner will reap the benefits of a reinvigorated sex life.

Be Careful!

Along these lines, I must add an important caveat: *draw the line at unprotected anal intercourse*. This practice is highly risky, even with the use of a condom. I have been surprised at how many heterosexual couples experiment with anal intercourse and how many enjoy it. Some are simply looking for new thrills. Others, interestingly, are looking for an alternative to vaginal intercourse due to religious or cultural reasons.

This issue has especially come to my attention in the last twenty years because people who practice anal sex, or are tempted to, have become increasingly concerned about HIV/AIDS. As a doctor, I must confirm that their concern is justified. It is no longer safe to think of anal intercourse as an occasional treat. HIV/AIDS is arguably the bubonic plague of the twenty-first century, and all studies indicate that a primary mode of transmission is through anal sex. The anus is particularly vulnerable to tears in the delicate tissue membrane, which expose the perianal blood vessels as a port of entry for the deadly retrovirus. Unprotected anal sex should be off limits on the basis of the HIV/AIDS risk alone. In addition, couples indulging in such practices should be aware that they bring other health risks as well. If the penis enters the rectum and comes in contact with fecal matter (which contains toxic bacteria, particularly E. coli), this can cause major infections in the prostate, bladder, kidneys, or blood. If the infection spreads to the bloodstream, it can result in sepsis, an infection that causes the body's immune system to attack the body's own organs and tissues. Sepsis can be fatal. In addition, if the penis is inserted into the rectum and then inserted into the vagina, it can contaminate the nearby urethra with fecal matter and cause a severe bladder infection in the female.

"Blow" Is Not an Accurate Description

Oral sex is another story entirely. For men who have been deprived of this pleasure, it could be just the thing to jump-start a tired sex life. The act itself has made many a reluctant penis as hard as a diamond. As we discussed earlier, the sucking action of the mouth literally creates a vacuum effect. This transmits a negative filling pressure to the blood vessels within the penile shaft, drawing blood into its channels. Psychologically, oral sex can also add an element of excitement to an intimate relationship. What a thrill for a man to experience his partner doing something so loving and gracious. For many men, it is just the thing to get them excited about sex and interested in exploring new sexual territory. In addition, many of my older patients have told me that the sucking action of oral sex is the *only* way they can obtain an erection firm enough for penetration, which is all the more reason to use oral sex as a way to improve your sex life.

Many women withhold this excellent form of stimulation from the men in their lives because they have a negative attitude toward it. Some women feel that it puts them in a subservient position. Some women have expressed to me that they oppose oral sex because they find it physically unpleasant if the man's penis touches the pharynx in the back of their throat. This can initiate the gag reflex. Some women have complained that oral sex is a one-way street—they are giving a man pleasure, but not receiving any back. All of these concerns are legitimate and understandable. But are they really *so* serious that they justify completely refusing to perform oral sex? There are many ways to position your body for oral sex—you do not have to be on your knees. Your man can easily position himself so he is stimulating you at the same time. Ask your man to refrain from thrusting his pelvis during oral sex because it makes you gag. He will surely oblige. A little practice should solve the problem.

It is important for any couple to establish and maintain a certain degree of sexual trust within an intimate relationship. All men should make a concerted effort to be aware of the physical effects of their actions on their partner. Superpotent men are keenly perceptive, particularly to the way their partners react during both oral sex and intercourse. All good sexual relationships entail giving and receiving. If you perform oral sex for your man, there is no harm in asking for something special in return.

Most women I meet in the context of my practice *enjoy* giving and receiving oral sex. They find the act erotic in and of itself, and many say it gives them a greater degree of control than other types of foreplay.

Many women take great pride in their ability to use their mouths and tongues creatively. "I love oral sex," a female colleague once told me, "because I'm damn good at it and because anything that gives my man pleasure pleases me."

If your partner is reluctant to perform oral sex, explain the physiology of why it gets a rise out of a penis. Allow your partner to express the reasons for her reservations. Try to assure your partner there is nothing dangerous, dirty, or sinful about it. If your partner had a bad experience with oral sex in the past, assure her that you care for her too much to hurt her in any way. At the same time, let your partner know that it would mean a lot to you personally. It just might add a whole new dimension to your sex lives.

A Time and Place for Everything

Gary was a young engineer who married his college sweetheart right after graduation. Soon after, they had a child. The marriage was going well in every respect, but things changed when the company Gary worked for was hit by a recession. The company fired a number of engineers, including Gary. When he told me he was having penis problems, I assumed it was because his self-esteem had taken a big blow as a result of the layoff. This is extremely common. Next to sexual issues, the areas that affect a man's self-image the most are those having to do with work and money. When a man suffers a financial setback or comes up short in his career goals, his masculinity takes a beating. This can manifest in penis failure. It is as if the mind says, "You messed up your career, you are less of a man, so you must also be inadequate sexually."

It is essential to understand the importance of this link between the health of your penis power and your ability to achieve success in other endeavors, like work and sports. It is very real and very powerful. In Gary's situation, it was not the whole problem. He had enough insight to realize that the layoff was an unfortunate turn of events that, in reality, had no bearing on his masculinity. At first, his sex life was not diminished. When his job hunting turned up nothing and the financial pressure mounted, he was forced to move his family into his parents' home. It was a temporary remedy while Gary explored job prospects in other parts of the country. It was during that period that he found his penis power dropping like the profits of his former company.

The reason? He was living in the house where he grew up, sleeping in the bedroom he used for eighteen years, and his parents were just a few yards away. This was the bedroom in which he self-consciously masturbated, hoping his parents would not barge in. This was the bedroom where he would sneak dates and nervously try to have sex before his parents got home. Next to his bed was the end table in which he once hid his *Playboy* collection. The associations were too strong. Just being there triggered all of the sexual anxieties of his adolescence. He was worried that his parents might overhear him and his wife making love. He worried that someone might walk in on them. Much of this was subconscious, of course, but all of that sexual anxiety was perfectly obvious to his penis.

When I suggested that the house might be the problem, Gary tested the hypothesis by checking into a motel with his wife. They had a sizzling weekend. As a result, he was able to laugh at the whole episode, and he quickly made different living arrangements.

Gary's situation is unusual, of course, but it is a good illustration of the relationship between *environment* and penis power. Location may not be as important in sex as it is in real estate, but it can play a major role in your ability to perform adequately. Noise, the wrong temperature, the possibility of being interrupted, lighting, negative associations, and every other little detail surrounding a sexual encounter can affect your penis performance. It is true that a superpotent man should rise to the challenge regardless of his environment, but everyone has specific preferences, and these really do make a difference. Some men like hard-driving rock 'n' roll while they romp with their lovers; some prefer violins. Some men like the sound of mellow jazz to get them in a romantic mood. Some men like the room totally dark; some like candlelight; and some like the lights on so they can see their naked partner. Some men are inhibited by the proximity of other people, and some find the danger of discovery a turnon. Some men like a cool room, and some like it steamy.

It is important for every man to recognize his own penis preferences. Does it perform better under certain conditions? What mood, setting, or location really puts you in a sexual state of mind? Why not do yourself the favor of arranging your sexual trysts to suit those preferences, or at least avoid situations that diminish your penis power? If you are not sure what your preferences may be, then do not be afraid to experiment until you find just what you are looking for. Once you and your trusted member discover the perfect balance, you will not be disappointed.

The Sweet Smell of Success

My patient Carl was a twenty-five-year-old actor with an enviable history of superpotent adventures. One day he fell madly in love. The sex was fantastic and so was the romance and emotional connection. After a whirlwind few weeks, the couple decided to move in together. Shortly thereafter, Carl started having erection failures. I thought for sure I knew what the problem was, as I had seen it before. "Carl," I said, "you're getting scared. Living with someone for the first time is terrifying. You feel trapped, my boy. You're afraid of losing your freedom, and it's expressing itself through your penis."

Carl was not so sure about that. He said he was happy to be living with someone. He wanted to continue doing so. He felt he was even *more* free because he had someone he loved to come home to. So I probed. Had anything changed since she moved in?

What was different? They had not had a fight. She had not started issuing demands or ultimatums. She was not trying to change him. She had not stopped wanting sex. He did not mention any of the other usual suspects. He then brought up something that hit home: she emitted a foul scent. The odor from her vagina had become very unpleasant to him. When they were dating, his girlfriend was very conscientious about her hygiene. Living together meant she did not always have the time or the motivation to tend to herself.

Carl had not considered this as a possible cause of his problem. A macho sort of guy, he thought nothing—let alone something seemingly as trivial as an odor—should interfere with his penis power. Like many men, he blamed himself. In fact, he found his girlfriend's scent so distasteful that no matter how aroused he was he became *unaroused* the moment she removed her panties. He did not have the heart to offer her an explanation.

I have examined thousands of women in my practice and have adopted the attitude of an environmental engineer when it comes to matters of hygiene. The vagina presents a number of unique conditions. Anatomically, it is a deep cavity with a relatively small opening and a large potential for expandable space within. It houses a variety of natural secretions and gets very little ventilation and hardly any light. This makes it a breeding ground for bacteria and yeast. Most women take pains to bathe thoroughly and wash regularly, especially when they anticipate having sex. It takes some modest effort for some women to keep their vaginas clean and pleasant-smelling. Many women do not always realize the effect that a strong, unpleasant scent can have on a man. Women should be especially aware of the effects of their body odor.

All women should make it a high priority to attend to vaginal hygiene, not only for reasons of general health but also especially so that it does not interfere with their romantic relationships. The same adherence to maintaining hygiene applies to men and their sexual apparatus as well. Men have just as much potential to emit bad odors from their penises as women do from their vaginas, and many women complain about just that. It behooves every superpotent man to pay extra-special care in keeping that very important appendage clean and pleasant-smelling.

I told Carl that, as difficult as it may be, it is important to *communicate* exactly how you feel if something is interfering with the health of a sexual relationship. If there is a problem, try to gently persuade your partner to be more attentive. With two adults in a good relationship, there is no reason not to suggest that they wash before getting intimate. You can even suggest taking a shower together before having sex, which is a great way to steam things up. Odors and discharges might not be a romantic topic of conversation, but if it is the second-most unpleasant aspect of sex, as my clinical experience has revealed, then it deserves to be discussed openly.

The Most Unpleasant Aspect of Sex

I know what you are thinking: if odor is in second place, what is in first? Sixty percent of the men whom I surveyed answered "an unresponsive partner."

What makes a penis the hardest is an *enthusiastic lover* in an equally conducive environment—a lover who is responsive and encourages what the man is doing. This is due to both the psychological lift a man gets from knowing that he is capable of exciting a desirable partner and the physiological response men have to stimulating their partner. Whatever the reason, the penis definitely responds to warmth, moisture, erotic sounds, tight embraces, and any other sign of satisfaction.

The opposite is also true. With a disinterested partner who has a cold body and a dry response, it takes an awfully strong penis to prevail.

Too many men take it personally when a lover fails to respond. They automatically assume it is their fault. They think there must be something wrong with *them*. The worst scenario is when a man, out of panic and fear, does not respond to the unresponsive partner.

This nonresponse usually leads to a downward spiraling, destructive chain of *nonreactions*. Ultimately, men who find themselves in this situation tend to think their penises have failed them. This is ridiculous. At some point in every man's sexual lifespan, he will have to deal with an unresponsive lover. There could be a number of reasons why your partner is not responding to you, many of which may have nothing to do with the actual act of sex at the moment.

It is important to be sensitive to the delicate clues your partner may be giving you and to communicate in an open, honest, and considerate way. Talk to your partner about her mood, and try to get her mind off of whatever preoccupation is distracting her from focusing on the erotic moment. If there is a conflict within the relationship, work it out before continuing to have sex. If you find yourself with an unresponsive partner, do your absolute best to excite her. Move slowly and explore the sensuality of the experience, paying close attention to the subtle body language of your lover. As a superpotent man, be persistent and diligent, delicate and precise. Learn everything you can about your partner's sexuality and preferences. What does she like? What turns her on? If necessary, make an effort to expand your sexual repertoire and learn some new "tricks." More importantly, do not blame yourself for what you cannot control. Do not pile any extra stress or anxiety onto your shoulders. Ultimately, if you pay attention to the delicate cues of an unresponsive partner and use every weapon in your sexual arsenal, you can make what was once a difficult situation a delightful walk in the park.

If you have tried your best and your partner is *still* unresponsive, you cannot let it affect your sexual self-esteem. You are not a failure if you have given it your best effort. Forgive yourself and move on. Your partner might have a serious hang-up that is beyond your ability to fix, or it might simply be a case of sexual incompatibility. It happens. There are matches made in hell, even for men of great penis power. Unfortunately, such incompatibility sometimes develops *after* a couple has been having satisfying sex. If that happens and you want the relationship to continue, by all means avail yourselves of whatever counseling or therapy is appropriate. The bottom line is to *just do something* before it becomes disastrous to both your emotional and sexual well-being.

It pains me to say that many of my patients are stuck with partners who do nothing to satisfy a man's desires, and those men feel there is nothing they can do about it. They shrug their shoulders and blame themselves. They sometimes run to their urologist for help. The reality is they do not need a urologist. All they need is to figure out how to remedy their situation or move on before their penises die a premature death.

Intimate Intimidation

There is an old joke that goes like this:

> There are two gates into heaven. Above one gate is a sign that reads, "Men Who Are Intimidated by Women." An endless line of men stretches out from this gate. Above the other gate is this sign: "Men Who Are Not Intimidated by Women." There is only one guy in line, and he is highly unattractive.
>
> Intrigued, Saint Peter walks up to this lone fellow and says, "Tell me, my son, what qualifies you to be in this line?"
>
> The man replies, "My wife told me to stand here."

Why does this joke get so many laughs? Because every man, even the strongest, most self-assured, and most independent superpotent man, at some time or another has felt intimidated by a woman. That is one of the deep secrets men carry. The strong ones laugh about it, the weak ones deny it. One thing is undeniable, however: a relentlessly intimidating partner is anathema to penis power.

What do I mean by intimidating? Most men like sexually aggressive partners who let them know what they want and are upfront about their desires. Every man has his own line that separates the kind of aggressiveness that arouses him from the negative kind that makes him want to run away. When aggressiveness is perceived as demanding or threatening, it can cause penis problems. Sometimes the aggressive gestures, words, and body language of some partners do not say, "I want you," but rather they scream, "Put up or shut up" or "I dare you to *try* to satisfy me."

Why are many men intimidated by demanding partners? Because aggressive and demanding lovers put pressure on these men to *perform*—and not just to perform, but to perform incredible feats of sexual wonder (at least that is what intimidated men think). If the demand is overtly challenging, it is like having someone command you military-style, "Get hard now!" That is tough for any man, especially if the intimidator is really saying, "I'm checking you out. I do not think you are man enough for me. And if you are not, I am going to let you know about it." Even if you have no previous history of penis weakness, a new set of overly aggressive demands can trigger the self-doubt that lurks deep within the psyche of almost every man: *Will* I satisfy you? *Can* I satisfy you? Will I measure up? What if I do not? And what happens once you start thinking those negative thoughts? Penis failure.

Never let yourself be intimidated. If you are with someone who has unrealistic expectations or puts too much pressure on you to perform, then communicate your feelings to him. Tell him how it makes you feel when he sets up unrealistic standards for you. If communication does not change his attitude, you may have to consider the possibility that he is not suitable as a partner for you. Intimidating lovers are not sexy. They are emasculating. Do not be fooled into thinking that a "real man" should meet crazy demands without blinking, or that failing to do so is a sign of personal inadequacy.

With regard to intimidation, many caring, good-hearted lovers intimidate men without even realizing it. One of the most common ways this can happen is exemplified by the following story about a patient of mine. He had been with his new girlfriend for six months, and everything was going well. One night they ran into her ex-boyfriend. He looked like a movie star and had the body of an all-pro halfback. My patient's girlfriend later told him about the ex-boyfriend. She said he was the best sex she had ever had. "He was unbelievable," she recalled. "He could go all night."

Her intention was innocent enough. She thought she was sharing an important part of her past with her boyfriend. The heart of her story was that the ex-boyfriend was really a jerk. His abusiveness was obscured by his sexual prowess. It had been an important lesson for her. But her innocent attempt to share an intimacy with her new boyfriend had a chilling effect on his penis power. He started wondering how his sexual performance compared to her ex-boyfriend's sexual performance. He grew fearful that he would lose his girlfriend because he might not match up to the ex-boyfriend's prowess. The result was an outbreak of penis weakness. After going over the situation with me one afternoon in my office, his predicament was clarified. His fear was all in his head. The girlfriend adored him. She was not comparing him sexually to the other man (at least she was smart enough to *say* she was not).

The bottom line is, whether real or imaginary, deliberate or unintentional, never *compare* your performance to some hypothetical or implied standard. All you can do is give each sexual encounter your best effort. As long as you do that, you should feel good about yourself. Your penis is what it is. Live with it and cherish it for what it is. What you *can* do is learn how to use it to the best of your capacity. Refuse to let yourself get caught up thinking of whom your lover might have been with in the past or if someone else may have been better at lovemaking than you. It does not matter if there are, or were, other men out there who can outperform you. If I were to compare myself to Tiger Woods every time I play golf, I would never tee off again. Just be yourself. Be confident in your performance ability, and never stop striving to become the best lover you can be.

When the Problem Is in Your Heart

Marty was a forty-seven-year-old business agent. He was in terrific physical shape and had acquired a reputation as a superpotent bachelor before he finally married Marilyn two years earlier. He told me, "I do not feel like making love to my wife lately, and when I do, I am . . . well, I am not the man I used to be. I want you to check my testosterone level."

I told him I would do the blood test to satisfy him, but I already knew the answer. Marty's testosterone was normal. Marty and I belonged to the same golf club. The previous weekend, I had seen Marty and his wife arguing heatedly in the parking lot. I asked him how things were between them. His answer was circumspect. I could tell from his body language that he was harboring a lot of anger.

"Go talk to Marilyn," I told him. "Straighten things out between you, and your penis will straighten out, too." I charged him an extra thirty-five cents for the psychiatric consultation and sent him on his way.

From my clinical experience, I long ago concluded that the greatest aphrodisiac ever invented is love itself. The opposite is also true: *the biggest enemy of sexual desire is hate*. For men in intimate relationships, nothing will make a penis slink away and hide as quickly as anger, hostility, or resentment toward a partner. If men fail to express their feelings and resolve their conflicts, the situation just gets worse. When they go through the motions of making love, their penises say, "I'm not getting hard for that—! Not after what was said about you and all those angry thoughts you have been thinking!"

My clinical studies have proven that diminished desire caused by anger will lead to penis weakness. Of all the extenuating circumstances that can affect a man's sexuality, the single most powerful factor is the nature of his relationship. If you are harboring animosity toward your partner, if you are rehashing angry feelings in your head without expressing them, if resentment has been accumulating in your heart so much that it obscures the love that brought you together, then how can it not affect what happens when you get into bed? This is why a man who aspires to great penis power should learn to deal effectively with his feelings and not let them contaminate his relationships.

With long-term partners especially, it is the heart that rules the penis. As time goes by, as the fires of passion diminish, and as the novelty of sex becomes routine, it is the emotions that guide the course of sexuality more than anything else. It is beyond the scope of this book, and of my professional expertise, to advise you on all the complexities of romantic and sexual relationships and the nuances of subtle emotions. What I can do is tell you what I tell my patients: *remove all the anger and resentment from your relationship and your love life will be strong and long-lasting.* Keep the love and affection alive. Do not take your partner for granted. Do not let your appreciation wane. Do not let petty animosities overshadow the qualities that have kept you together.

Two mature people with a strong commitment have the greatest potential for mutually satisfying sex. This does not mean that problems still will not arise. Every relationship has conflicts: sex, money, children, in-laws, and the thousand annoyances that make up everyday life. You must be aware that every conflict affects your penis. You also have to be aware that the most effective response to a conflict is to work things out in a healthy and effective way. Do everything in your power to resolve those difficulties in a forthright and honest manner.

Communicate. If you cannot do it on your own, then by all means find a counselor or a friend who can help you. Get your feelings out in the open. That does not just mean venting your emotions or allowing your feelings to come out in negative and hurtful ways. It means truly discussing the issues in an atmosphere of fairness and mutual respect where each party listens, as well as speaks.

A superpotent man is not afraid to show his vulnerability. If he is angry, it is because he has been hurt or offended. A superpotent man knows it is best to vent his negative feelings rather than hold them in and explode at some inopportune moment. If your relationship is built on a solid foundation, then your partner will respond with equally genuine feelings. When that happens, the love you have buried beneath your anger has a good chance of rising to the surface, and your penis is likely to rise with it.

As Old as You Feel: The Life Story of the Penis

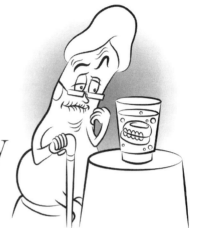

Is it not strange that desire should so many years outlive performance?" Shakespeare eloquently and perceptively once noted.[1] It might seem strange to men whose penis power appears to diminish with age, but it is certainly not strange to a urologist. Of all the circumstances that affect the functioning of a penis, the most predictable is the normal, inevitable process of aging.

By far, the most frequent complaint I hear is a variation on the following: "Something's wrong, Doc. I am not the man I used to be." What men usually mean when they say that is that they do not have the same level of *sexual desire* they used to have, it takes longer to get an erection, it takes longer to ejaculate, it takes longer to get aroused again after they make love, and their erections are not as firm, or some of the above or all of the above. These are all predictable changes that occur as men get older. They happen at different times to different men, but they happen to every man who lives long enough.

Problems arise with either of two responses to the aging process: (1) the patient does not realize that such changes are normal, so he concludes that he has a medical or psychological problem; or (2) he *does* know that these developments are typical and concludes that he is hopelessly over the hill. Either conclusion is erroneous and detrimental to a man's overall happiness and to his penis health in particular.

A typical example of the first kind of man is a colleague of mine. A radiologist approaching his fiftieth birthday, he had always been a man of superpotency and excellent general fitness. Noticing that he was getting cramps in his legs while running, he saw an internist. The diagnosis was claudication, a condition characterized by cramping of the leg muscles while exercising. This is caused by diminished blood flow. Claudication is usually the result of arteriosclerotic plaque blocking the arteries supplying blood to the legs. The radiologist concluded that if the blood flow in his legs had become impeded, the same might also be true of the blood supply to his penis. This was the explanation for which my colleague had been searching. He had been alarmed for some time by a decline in his penis power. His ego had prevented him from saying anything to me in the past, but now that he was sure it was a medical problem, he opened up. He had his condition evaluated by a vascular surgeon and then came to me for treatment.

After a complete uro-vascular profile, I was able to say without reservation that the blood flow to his penis was nearly as good as it was when he was thirty. I suggested that perhaps a little help from vasoactive pills (e.g., Viagra, Levitra, Cialis) would be the answer. It turned out his penis power was still at a very high level, but his erections were not as firm as they used to be. That was the problem. When he compared the firmness of his erection to what it was five or ten years earlier, he was clearly losing ground. I asked him, "Do you run as far as you did at twenty-five? Can you jump as high? Can you lift as much weight? Can you do as many push-ups? Can you dance until dawn? You do not expect to do those things at your age. You know what happens to our bodies as we age. That is why athletes retire in their thirties. How, then, do you expect your penis to be as firm at age fifty as it was at age twenty?"

The other response to aging is typified by the countless men who resign themselves to a sexless life. They are often worn out, ailing, cynical, and prone to complaining about life in general. Some enter retirement and lose their enthusiasm and joy for living. Many men experience a slight loss of memory or hearing as they age. They begin to interpret changes in their sexuality as a sign of impending death. They put their penises out to pasture without even a gold watch or a ceremony. What a sad waste of penis power!

The key point to remember is this: as you age, you do not lose penis power, and your penis performance does not become inferior. It simply changes. It becomes different. Unless you have a legitimate medical disorder that interferes with your penis functioning, you can be as superpotent at eighty as you were at twenty. It is essential to understand the changes that come about with aging, accept them gracefully, adjust your attitude, and make the most of what you have. It is all relative, and it is all in your head—your *big head* that is.

Penis Passages

To understand what happens to the penis as men age, we must first examine the ways in which the penis evolves from birth through adulthood.

From birth until puberty, the penis is basically a conduit for urine. The mechanism of erection, however, is present even before birth. All male children, including infants, get erections. They are involuntary and not associated with anything sexual. These childhood erections occur due to nerve stimulation and can be caused by a full bladder or rubbing the penis with a towel after bathing.

Then comes puberty. Peculiar things start happening. The testicles have developed to the point where they produce enough circulating testosterone to alter the size and appearance of certain body parts. At this stage, a boy develops *secondary sexual characteristics*, including facial, underarm, and pubic hair, a deeper voice, adult-size genitalia, and the ability to ejaculate. Suddenly, the penis is a wonderful novelty! Adolescents cannot play with theirs enough. Simply looking at a sexy picture or a girl's legs can stimulate the young penis to a full erection. Teens realize they can masturbate and inevitably discover that it can be even nicer with a partner.

Typically, when a boy reaches his late teens, he becomes sexually obsessed. His level of desire, the ease with which he becomes aroused, and his capacity for frequent sex are astounding. Dominated by hormones, physically fit, and not yet burdened by adult responsibilities, the teenage male is a walking erection, capable of getting one at any time with little or no provocation and ejaculating five or six times a day! At no time does the penis rule the brain more than it does in adolescence. I am reminded of the time a professor of mine brought down the house with a cogent observation about young men in college. Princeton was not yet coed when I was an undergraduate, so the auditorium was filled with a few hundred male freshmen in a philosophy survey course. The professor looked over the students and said, "All of you guys out there with such brilliant minds have this piece of meat hanging between your legs. These days, your whole life is fixed on that piece of beef. It's all you think about, day and night. If there were any way to channel the mental energy focused on your collective dicks into a more productive intellectual plane, I might find a Nobel laureate out there, and surely most of you would go through college Phi Beta Kappa and summa cum laude while saving a hell of a lot of energy in the process!" The room roared with laughter, and the professor reveled in his accurate depiction of the power of the penis on the mind of an adolescent male.

The Early Years

The penis problems that I treat in patients in their late teens and early twenties are typically those associated with hypersensitivity. The young man who is unsure of himself and is worried about whether he is as normal or as virile as his friends might lose his perpetual erection at precisely the wrong moment because of sheer nervousness. More typical is the problem of premature ejaculation. As discussed in chapter 3, the adolescent penis is extremely sensitive, the volume of semen produced is higher than at any other stage of life, and the young man usually has not had enough experience to develop self-control. He might ejaculate before penetration or immediately thereafter. This could be embarrassing enough to make a young man shy away from sex permanently. If only the lad knew how typical this was!

The solution for most young men is simply to have more frequent ejaculations. (In this age of AIDS, I must add a cautionary note: frequent sex should not be regarded as synonymous with indiscriminate sex.) For men in their late teens and early twenties, the refractory period can be as short as a few minutes. If you ejaculated prematurely the first time, the next time you will last longer simply because there is less fluid in your seminal vesicles and less physiological urgency to release it. It requires a higher level of stimulation over a longer period of time to get through the excitatory phase to when the reflex of ejaculation occurs. I'll explain more about premature ejaculation later.

In spite of these facts, there is a surprisingly large number of men with penis weakness in their early to late twenties. It almost never stems from something physical, even though, medically speaking, the "peak" of sexuality might have been passed at age nineteen or twenty. It seems to have more to do with the *stage* of life they have now entered. The young men in this group are usually out of school and no longer in a safe and predictable environment where their stature revolves around popularity issues. They are no longer protected by their parents. They are suddenly dealing with the harsher realities of life and making "grown-up" decisions. The "big man on campus" is now the "little man" in the office. The star student now has to pass tests that are not on paper and are not multiple choice. The girls he picked up in classrooms and fraternity houses are now young women with mature needs and demands of their own. The young man may find himself in a real relationship for the first time, along with the complexity and confusion that comes with it. For the first time, he is working long, hard hours. He usually feels exhausted by Friday. Work pressures and strain are impinging upon him. These negative forces are not easily brushed aside.

All of this often leads to a high level of *stress*. For someone without the skills, seasoning, or maturity to deal with it, the result can be devastating. Most young men have not yet developed the ability to *compartmentalize* their lives. Such pressures can often cause a young man to question his masculine identity. A serious case of self-doubt can occur and inevitably lead to unwanted penis consequences.

Is It Ageless?

Then come other changes. These changes evolve from the peak period of sexuality until your penis is laid to rest with your other organs at life's end. Interestingly, these changes will not be seen in the penis itself. Agelessness is one of the most remarkable aspects of the penis, and yet another paradox. The penis undergoes virtually *no change in size or appearance as you age*. While your other organs degenerate, your skin wrinkles, your waistline expands, your hair gets gray, and your scalp starts to show through, your aging penis continues to look nearly the same as it always did. If you were to compare an unaltered photograph of a twenty-year-old erect penis side by side with an eighty-year old erect penis, you would not be able to tell the difference! The same is more or less true of flaccid penises, although the trained eye of a urologist might discern a subtle difference. In the elderly penis, there is some relaxation of the suspensory ligaments (located just under the pubic bone), which gives the impression that the penis has lengthened. This is more illusory than real; the penis is not really longer, it is just drooping a bit. Conversely, there is no *shrinkage* of the penis with age, as many men fear. Remember, the length and width of the erect penis are dictated by the size of the corpora cavernosa, the tubular structures that fill with blood in the erect state. That does not change once a man reaches maturity.

What does change with age is how the penis behaves. The first thing older men notice is that it takes longer to get an erection. This might start happening to men during their twenties. It might happen so gradually that it is not even noticed until they approach middle age. Much depends on the kinds of relationships they have and the frequency of their sexual activity. At some point, men discover that it takes *more* stimulation to get them hard. Once your testosterone levels diminish with age, fantasies are no longer enough; the mere sight of a sexy body might not do it, nor even heated foreplay. It might require a little more direct stimulation from your partner. As I previously noted, many older men can only get an erection from the vacuum effect of oral sex and the psychological aspects associated with that sexual act.

As you age, you might also notice that your erections are not always as rigid as a steel rod like they were during your teenage years. Sometimes they are only half-hard or semirigid until added stimulation hopefully brings them to full strength. This, too, is normal, but men often greet this phenomenon with panic, recalling the days when they seemed to spend half of their time concealing their erections.

The same is true of the refractory period. It is a well-documented urologic fact that the amount of time it takes to recover after an ejaculation increases in proportion to a man's age and the volume of the ejaculate decreases. When a man reaches his fifties and six-ties, the refractory period might be as long as twenty-four hours, even with direct stimulation. At age eighty, it might be one week. Men also notice that the ejaculation itself feels less and less explo-sive as they age; the semen leaks out rather than being forcefully expelled. Orgasms might also feel less intense. All of this is a nor-mal part of the aging process. You should anticipate these changes and greet them without bitterness or alarm.

The good news is that with age comes increased experience, wisdom, and seasoning, which should be a huge boon to your sex life. There is an old story that illustrates this fact with a bit of hu-mor. Two bulls, an old bull and a really young bull, are roaming the plains of Wyoming. They come upon a ridge overlooking a valley filled with thirty grazing cows, and the young bull jumps up and down with excitement, shouting, "Let's *run* down this hill as fast as we can and screw us a few cows!" The old bull, surveying the situa-tion, turns ever so calmly to his young companion and says, "Son, how about we mosey on down there *real slow* and screw them *all*!"

The point of this story is that as you age, your body may not be as flexible as it once was, your sex drive may diminish, and your erec-tions may not be as firm, but your wisdom and sexual insight can be used to your advantage. Do not panic if it takes a little longer to get erect. On the contrary, you and your partner can enjoy the extra foreplay required to get you ready. Do not feel let down if you can-not go at it a second or third time without a long rest—this does not signify a decline in your manhood. Focus your attention instead on getting the absolute most out of the intercourse you can handle. Do not be let down if your ejaculations are not as volcanic as they once were—you can still enjoy the pleasure of orgasm well into old age.

Sex does not get less enjoyable with age or become in any way inferior. It just becomes *different*. Sex can be better than ever if you have the right attitude. Not only do you naturally acquire greater ejaculatory control, but if you have been paying attention over the years, you should also have learned a great deal about women in general, and your partner in particular. You should have learned tricks for arousing and satisfying the person with whom you share your bed, and vice versa.

One thing you may have to do as you age, especially when you reach your sixties and seventies, is adjust your *style* of lovemaking. Your penis might look as young as ever, but the rest of you has aged. You might have more control over when you ejaculate, but your arms might not be strong enough to support you for as long as they used to do. The muscles in your back and legs might tire quickly, and your joints and ligaments might not be as flexible. This may mean you have to rest or change positions more often. You might have to try different positions entirely.

The fact that physical fitness is an important aspect of maintaining sexual strength should encourage you to maintain a healthy lifestyle. You should make it a priority now to improve your overall health and fitness with a healthy diet and a vigorous exercise regimen, before the effects of aging begin to ravage your body. If you keep a positive attitude, you will find all of this a challenge, not a burden.

Another change occurs with age, and this one should be viewed as a bonus: it takes *longer* to reach orgasm. As the old joke from the old guy goes, "It takes all night to do what I used to do all night long." But this is not a problem, especially if you found it difficult to control your ejaculations in the past. Young men who were quick on the trigger find their sex lives far more satisfying when they reach the age when delaying orgasm is no longer a chore but a natural process. If your partner is a woman, she may even get more pleasure because it is usually easier to bring a woman to orgasm with prolonged intercourse than with quick encounters. The more satisfied your partner is, the more aroused *you* will be.

For some men, the problem might be that it takes *too* long to ejaculate in general, and not just as they age. This is usually associated with a reduced level of sensitivity in the penis or a habitual mind-set that views prolonged sex as the only way to achieve orgasm, or both. Because some partners who are otherwise willing may find prolonged sex irritating, painful, or unpleasant, I recommend prolonging foreplay, trying new positions, and otherwise addressing whatever issues may be causing the problem. Some men believe they have to perform a sexual marathon to please their partners. This belief can be problematic, especially in situations where men *assume* that what they want for themselves is compatible with their partners' needs. Regardless of the scenario, it is crucial for men to make the appropriate adjustments to accommodate their partners' comfort level. Communication, awareness, and consideration are the best triad to navigate the intricate workings of a sexual relationship, especially as you age.

When the Going Gets Tough: Male Menopause and TRT

Getting old is not for wimps. It is an undeniable fact that as we age, we can no longer run as fast, jump as high, or dance all night long the way we used to do. Similar to what happens to women during menopause, for men over forty, testosterone levels start to fall at an average of about 1 percent per year. As indestructible teenagers, it was testosterone that helped build our muscles and develop strong bones. As young men, record-setting levels of testosterone made us heroes on the gridiron on a sunny, Saturday afternoon, boosted our energy levels to allow "all-nighters" with ease, and propelled our foolish actions with the false belief that our youthful bodies could scale an unattainable mountaintop or perhaps even leap from a helicopter without a parachute and land on our toes with the grace of a ballet dancer.

As urologists learn more about the role of testosterone in the physical and mental development of young men in their prime, we are also studying the role of testosterone in the aging body. With this in mind, testosterone replacement therapy (TRT) has been promoted in the print media and television, and especially over the Internet as the solution to the male equivalent of female menopause (in men, it is known as andropause). TRT brings with it the promise that it will improve a man's libido, increase muscle mass, eliminate cognitive deficiencies, elevate mood, and bolster bone density.

Progressive testosterone (androgen) deficiency in aging men has led to a syndrome known as hypogonadism, which can manifest in osteoporosis (loss of bone density), decreased libido, erectile dysfunction, and mood changes (i.e., the "grumpy old man syndrome"). In addition, hypogonadism causes muscles to become flabby and decrease in size, leaving men with the dreaded middle-age paunch. Hypogonadism has become widely recognized over the past ten years. As a result, physicians have increased the number of testosterone replacement prescriptions at an enormous rate. Pharmaceutical statistics indicate a 500 percent increase in the use of testosterone products in the elderly and middle-aged population, promoting the hopes of turning potbellies into lean six-packs, fragile bones into pillars of strength, and grumpy old men into enthusiastic Lotharios.

Who Needs Testosterone Replacement?

In order for a physician to determine if a patient needs testosterone replacement therapy (TRT), blood levels of testosterone must be assessed. Some important numbers should be kept in mind when measuring serum testosterone: the accepted low limit for normal adult men is a testosterone level of at least 200 ng/dl (nanograms per deciliter). If a man's serum testosterone is below 200 ng/dl, TRT is recommended. If a man's serum testosterone level falls between 200 and 400 ng/dl, the risk-to-benefit ratio of TRT and its attendant hazards, which I will discuss below, must be considered. This range of testosterone level is considered a *grey zone* for TRT. Therefore, all of the potential risks of TRT must be discussed between the patient and his doctor. For serum testosterone levels of greater than 400 ng/dl, not only is there *no benefit* to TRT, but there is also considerable risk involved. Men who are experiencing some of the symptoms of andropause should consult a physician, have their serum testosterone checked, and determine how best to proceed with treatment, if any.

Good News, but at a Price

No discussion of TRT would be complete unless we weighed the risks against the benefits. First, the long-term effects of TRT are not well defined. The main areas of concern for me are cardiovascular and prostate problems, both of which are commonly associated in men with diminished testosterone levels. Cardiologists have noted that the increased incidence of coronary artery disease in men, compared with women, may be testosterone-dependent. It has been found that men receiving long-term TRT have significant changes in their lipid profiles. These changes directly affect cardiovascular health. Unfortunately, TRT lowers the beneficial cholesterol (high density lipids, or HDL) widely recognized for its role in protecting against coronary artery disease. This is bad. The good news is that TRT *also* lowers the bad cholesterol (low density lipids, or LDL) responsible for blocking coronary arteries. It is encouraging that these effects on the lipid profile may be minimal when TRT maintains a serum testosterone level below 400 ng/dl. However, the cardiac risks increase dramatically when TRT is taken to abusive or supra-physiological levels above 500 ng/dl.

Another effect of TRT is increased production of red blood cells. This increase causes a hypercoagulation state of the blood, causing a thickening that may increase the potential for a stroke or heart attack. This is especially true in smokers, who already have an increased circulating red blood cell volume. Therefore, I do not recommend TRT that raises serum testosterone above 400 ng/dl. Having a healthy heart and healthy arteries should not be compromised by the desire to get a slender waistline or bodybuilder muscles.

If you start TRT, do not exceed the recommended dosage in an attempt to radically change your physical appearance. To the aging man who longs for that youthful body that is beginning to disappear, my advice is to modify your diet, maintain a healthy exercise routine, and accept the realities of aging—a reality that sometimes brings with it a little paunch.

The second most important issue surrounding the risks of TRT is understanding its impact on prostate disease. It is well known that TRT *does not* induce the development of prostate cancer. What it can do, however, is cause rapid and potentially catastrophic growth of an unrecognized prostate cancer. There is no evidence that TRT can create prostate cancers. However, if there is even a tiny focus of cancerous cells in an otherwise benign prostate, TRT can encourage these cells to grow explosively. This can potentially become life-threatening. In my clinical experience, the incidence of prostate cancer in patients who have been on TRT for at least six months is no more than the rate of prostate cancer among men not taking testosterone. The take-home message here is if a man is receiving TRT, his doctor should be meticulously monitoring his prostate health with a periodic digital rectal examination (DRE), cancer screening blood tests (i.e., the PSA test), and prostatic ultrasonography.

With the overwhelming media blitz promoting treatment for male andropause, my patients are asking if TRT is safe and if I recommend it. In my judgment, it is safe to use TRT, and it is clearly beneficial in *symptomatic* men with a serum testosterone level of less than 200 ng/dl. In men whose serum testosterone is greater than 400 ng/dl, it is *unacceptable*. Ultimately, testosterone replacement therapy remains a calculated risk for men over forty, and unfortunately for some men, youthful fantasies must take a back seat to the realities of medical science.

If TRT is suitable for you as a patient, then there are some choices to be made. Unfortunately, all oral preparations of testosterone have been abandoned in the United States because of severe liver toxicity. An acceptable alternative for TRT is intramuscular injection. This has considerable appeal because it is relatively inexpensive. The downside is that dosing is intermittent, which means that the highest levels of serum testosterone are achieved shortly after the injection. Toward the end of the cycle, which usually lasts two to three weeks, the blood level of serum testosterone has diminished to pretreatment levels. Therefore, the effect of the circulating testosterone is variable with high peaks and deep valleys. There are implantable testosterone pellets that are also available. These have the advantage of producing a more stable level of serum testosterone. This treatment modality is expensive and cumbersome, and complications can include unanticipated pellet extrusion, which is uncomfortable.

Over the past several years, an exciting new treatment modality for TRT known as transdermal application has been developed. Transdermal preparations allow the testosterone to be applied directly to the skin with a patch or a gel. This allows absorption to occur through the skin and into the bloodstream, resulting in a normal, steady, and effective level of circulating serum testosterone over a twenty-four-hour period. The transdermal patches are less desirable than the gel. The patches often cause skin irritation, known as contact dermatitis. Transdermal gel, either Testim 1 percent or Androgel, is applied on a non-hair-bearing surface. Testosterone gels are relatively expensive when compared to the cost per month for injectable testosterone. If you need testosterone replacement therapy, your best choice is to find a treatment modality that suits both your physical and financial needs. The results of TRT for symptomatic men are quite remarkable and will improve many of the physical effects associated with the toughest part of life—getting old.

Young at Heart, Young in Person

I cannot reiterate this point enough: *attitude* is the key to penis longevity. My superpotent patients tell me that sex gives them as much joy at seventy as it did at twenty. Some say it is even better! From my clinical experience, I have concluded that equal pleasure can be obtained from occasional, prolonged intercourse with one orgasm as with frequent, rapid intercourse with multiple orgasms.

Many men give up their sex lives as soon as they start identifying themselves as "old," especially once they retire. The idea that retirement equals nirvana is an unfortunate myth perpetrated in our modern culture. I have observed in my practice that retirement can lead to inertia, boredom, and stagnation. Many of my older patients, even those who are wealthy, choose not to retire. They may cut back their hours and delegate a lot of responsibility to others, but they remain active, both in work and in play. These individuals tend to be my healthiest, most superpotent patients. They live longer, and the quality of their lives seems better than those who stop challenging themselves and throw in the towel for retirement. Do not voluntarily retire your penis unless you are forced to by circumstances beyond your control, such as a serious illness.

Until recently, our society's image of aging usually excluded sex. It had been considered unseemly for older people to *talk* about it, much less *do* it. I know elderly people who have to sneak around to have sex just as they did when they were teenagers because they know it will be frowned upon by their peers and especially by their own children. Other older people stop having sex altogether because they buy into the notion that they are *supposed* to give up sex. They suppress their sexuality because it somehow seems inappropriate to express it.

It is my hope that the generation I now see entering their senior years challenges all of that. They deserve active, healthy sex lives as long as they remain physically fit. It will not harm them unless they try to do things their muscles and joints are too weak to manage or they overextend themselves to the point of exhaustion. Do not expect to do at fifty what you could do at forty, or do at sixty what you could do at fifty, and so on. Adjust your sexual activities as your body changes, just as you adjust other activities. Look upon the adjustment as both a new challenge and a new opportunity. As you age, learn to use your mind and imagination to make up in creativity what you may lack in physical strength.

As long as you are able to breathe, move your extremities, maintain relative control over your bodily functions, remain alert enough to identify the date and day of the week, and sustain a positive mental outlook, you can continue to exercise your penis power indefinitely. You can help stay superpotent as you age by maintaining good overall health habits: exercising regularly; minimizing your consumption of fat and cholesterol; controlling your weight; refraining from smoking, excessive drinking, and drugs; watching your blood pressure; and seeing your physician regularly. If you stay physically fit and mentally alert, you can remain sexually active as long as you have the urge.

Most importantly, *do not think old*! Your body may produce less testosterone; your blood vessels may become partially obstructed and diminish blood flow to the penis; and your muscles and joints may begin to deteriorate. But if your mind is still strong, your penis can be strong, too. The key is not to lament what you have lost. Be grateful for what you still have, and make the most of it. Age is not a deterrent to a superpotent man. Rather, it is a challenge and an opportunity. Think of yourself as a singer whose voice is not as powerful as it once was, but who more than makes up for it with phrasing, feeling, and subtlety. Think of yourself as an athlete or dancer whose legs are no longer as strong as oaks but who performs with added grace shaped by the wisdom that comes with experience. If you keep your enthusiasm, you can compensate for, or even delay, the effects of aging.

If you have penis power, you are young no matter what your age may be. The strenuous use of your penis will sharpen your mind, exalt your soul, and keep you feeling vigorous. In short, you do not stop having sex because you get old, *you get old because you stop having sex*!

In many ways, your later years should be the golden years for your sexuality. You do not have to get up and go to the office in the morning, you do not have to worry as much about kids and bills, you have less daily stress and fewer pressures, you have more privacy, you have more time, and you can afford the luxury of patience. This is an opportunity for a superpotent man to make the most of his penis power.

Andropause versus Menopause

It is also important to acknowledge that as long-term couples age, significant changes occur in both partners. As women experience menopause, their sexuality goes through extreme changes. For the most part, postmenopausal women have a *decreased* sex drive and are not as interested in sex as they may have been in the past. This is due largely to the marked decrease in estrogen (which is analogous to testosterone) that accompanies menopause, as well as the psychological effects of an aging body (i.e., loss of hair, changes in physical appearance, and often extreme emotional fluctuations). Many women become depressed during menopause. A caring partner must go the extra mile to be sensitive to these changes. Compassion and patience must abound, both inside and outside of the bedroom.

In many aging couples, the lack of vaginal lubrication can become a major obstacle for sex. When estrogen levels start to fall, it becomes increasingly difficult for the vagina to lubricate itself. Topical estrogen or the use of oils can help in maintaining vaginal lubrication. A variety of lubricants can be used effectively and safely. Postmenopausal women have a far greater *disinterest* in sex than men experiencing andropause. For this reason, the superpotent man must adjust his expectations and learn how to work around the effects of aging on his partner's body. Talking candidly to your partner about these changes is the best way to find a solution for maintaining a healthy sex life. Above all, do not turn your back on your lifelong partner for a younger, more responsive lover. Beware of the "hard dick syndrome": a young, sexy lover might make you feel like a stud, but you may realize very quickly that sacrificing the friendship, intimacy, and bond of a long-term relationship might not be worth the quick fix of a young lover.

Sex is not only safe for older couples, it is also good for them. It maintains overall physical strength, cardiovascular health, and most of all, it keeps them invigorated. Your penis is there to serve you from puberty to old age. Do not give up on your penis, and it will not give up on you.

Penis Posterity

One good reason to be optimistic about the longevity of your penis power is that medical science is capable of helping you, even if aging has reduced the capacity of your body. We know the single most common cause of erectile dysfunction with aging is arteriosclerosis, the abnormal thickening and hardening of the arterial walls. This can restrict the blood flow to the penis and keep it from getting firm enough to penetrate. If a patient with arteriosclerosis is motivated, there are the many treatments we have discussed that can help him, which include prosthetic implants, vacuum erection devices (VEDs), self-injectable vasoactive drugs such as papaverine and prostaglandin-E, and the oral agents (Viagra, Cialis, Levitra). Certain drugs used for lowering cholesterol can also be helpful.

With respect to the use of prosthetic devices and injectable medications, I want to again make an important distinction between the type of patients for whom I do and do not recommend such treatments. A typically acceptable candidate is the man who is suffering from the "leisure world syndrome." He is often a widower in his late sixties or seventies. He starts to meet older women in a social context, and he begins to date. To his surprise, these women expect a level of sexual activity that he did not anticipate. He is not necessarily able to handle the challenge. This type of patient was usually not very sexually active in the latter years of his marriage. This was perhaps due to his wife's illness, his own reduced capacity due to impaired blood flow, or perhaps it was simply due to the diminished desire that accompanies long marriages. Now, for the first time in years, when he is called upon to perform, he *wants* to satisfy his new companion, but he is nervous or embarrassed. He feels like he is less of a man.

If such a patient is in otherwise good physical condition, I aggressively offer solutions and encourage him to take advantage of them. This kind of patient is a legitimate candidate for a prosthetic implant or vasoactive injections, but generally only if he has not responded well to the oral medications (i.e., Viagra, Cialis, Levitra).

On the other end of the spectrum is an aging man who has been married for many years to the same woman. The couple has had a fulfilling life together and remain very much in love, even though their sex life has diminished, perhaps to the point of total inactivity. When they do attempt to have sex, the man finds he is incapable of getting an erection. In a burst of forgotten youth, he decides he wants his old sex life back again and comes to me for help. If I feel he is seeking treatment in the vain hope that it will restore his youthful vigor and virility, I do not encourage implants or vasoactive injections. If the marriage has already adjusted to the absence of sex, these aggressive treatments are not advised. I have found that, once the novelty wears off, this type of patient usually discontinues using the devices. Many a wife has told me that her husband used the prosthesis or self-injection a few times and then stopped. Each case has to be evaluated on an individual basis, preferably with the partner involved in the decision. Treatment has done much good for some marriages of fifty years and longer.

Sex in the New Millennium

I would like to close this chapter on aging with a prediction. Based on my clinical experience and my understanding of current research, I am convinced that the future bodes well for the sex lives of people now entering their senior years and even better for those now middle-aged. I base this prediction on the burgeoning cultural view that the elderly can be active and fulfilled, even when it comes to sex. This is in addition to the amazing progress that has been made in extending the capacities of other bodily functions. The upper limits of what the body can do have been continuously broadened. In sports, what were once considered insurmountable barriers, such as the four-minute mile and the seven-foot high jump, are all now accomplished routinely. The peak years of athletes have been dramatically extended through unique conditioning procedures, nutritional advances, and medical science. There is no reason why the years of active sexuality cannot be similarly extended. There is no reason why penis power cannot continue to grow in aging men.

In this new century, people will be sexually active into their nineties! For one thing, lifespan will continue to increase. Impressive medical advancements, healthier lifestyles, and new discoveries in the field of genetics will continue. This research holds the promise to prolong life through drugs and genetic engineering. I predict that the *quality* of life in old age will improve geometrically. The elderly are far more vital and far more dynamic than ever before. In addition, society's attitude toward sex and the elderly is becoming more permissive. It will no doubt become far more acceptable to be sexually active into old age, a trend that will probably accelerate as the generation that came of age during the sexual revolution approaches seniority. For men who are young now, the golden years will truly provide the opportunity for the enjoyable, leisurely exercise of penis power, as long as they are willing to use it.

Chapter 10

Sexually Transmitted Diseases

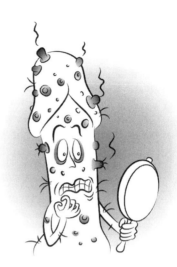

L et us hold off for a minute on what should be your primary concern—HIV/AIDS—and talk about the sexually transmitted diseases (STDs) that have faded from the spotlight over the past few years, but are still very much with us. STDs remain a major public health challenge throughout the world today. While significant progress has been made in preventing, diagnosing, and treating certain STDs, the Centers for Disease Control and Prevention (CDC) estimates that nineteen million new infections occur each year in the United States alone. In Los Angeles County over a period of four years, the county saw a 58 percent increase in the reported rate of infection for primary and secondary syphilis and a 32 percent increase in gonorrhea.[1] The country as a whole continues to have a high incidence of genital herpes and chlamydia. The good news is that, when diagnosed properly, most STD infections can be treated. In many cases, once the symptoms are gone, they have no deleterious effect on penis power. Let us look at the various STDs.

Chlamydia: Silent but Troublesome

Chlamydia remains the most commonly reported infectious disease in the United States. It is estimated there are nearly 2.8 million new cases of chlamydia each year.[2] Chlamydia is a bacterial infection that can easily be cured with antibiotics. It is usually asymptomatic, meaning it rarely shows or produces indications of a disease or medical condition; therefore it often goes undiagnosed. Untreated, it can cause severe health consequences for women, including pelvic inflammatory disease (PID) and ectopic pregnancy. *Ectopic* means "out of place." In an ectopic pregnancy, a fertilized egg is implanted outside the uterus. The egg settles in the fallopian tubes more than 95 percent of the time. An ectopic pregnancy can cause fetal death and present grave dangers for the mother. The fallopian tubes can only expand about one inch. When the fetus surpasses this size, tubular rupture ensues and the baby is miscarried. This places the mother at extreme risk. Permanent damage to her reproductive organs is probable.

In addition, many gynecologists report that chlamydia is one of the leading causes of infertility in women. Even more alarming is the fact that women infected with chlamydia are up to five times more likely to become infected with HIV, if exposed. The chlamydia organism is responsible for nearly 40 percent of all recurring vaginal infections that do not respond to traditional treatment. In men, it can cause epididymitis, an inflammation or infection of the epididymis (a duct located on the posterior surface of the testicle), resulting in pain and swelling of the testicle. Chlamydia can also cause nonspecific urethritis, an inflammation of the male urethra. Often there are no symptoms, but the infection can still be transmitted. If symptoms do develop, they are likely to include a watery discharge and burning when you urinate. A simple urine test can detect chlamydia. The organism can then be effectively treated with antibiotics.

Gonorrhea: This Clap Is Not a Cheer

The second most reported genital infectious disease in the United States is gonorrhea, often called the "clap." The nickname of the clap refers to a treatment that used to clear the blockage in the urethra from gonorrhea pus where the penis would be "clapped" on both sides simultaneously. This primitive treatment for gonorrhea is not used today; however, the nomenclature remains.

With the advent of penicillin, to which gonorrhea is extremely sensitive, the disease has been on a steady rate of decline since 1941. From 1975 to 2004, the rate declined 76 percent, to the lowest recorded level since reporting began. However, it remains a highly infectious disease and a major global health problem. An infected patient usually comes in with a yellowish and pus-like discharge from the penis. While gonorrhea is easily cured, untreated cases can lead to serious health problems. Among women, gonorrhea, like Chlamydia, is a major cause of pelvic inflammatory disease (PID).

In men, untreated gonorrhea can cause chronic epididymitis and, more significantly, can involve the urethra and the prostate, causing severe scarring and lifelong strictures (abnormal narrowing in the urethra). Like chlamydia, studies suggest that the presence of gonorrhea makes an individual three to five times more likely to acquire HIV, if exposed. Fortunately, gonorrhea can usually be cured with oral or injected antibiotics. Drug resistance, however, is becoming an increasingly important concern in treatment and prevention. Resistance is especially worrisome among men who have sex with men, where resistance is eight times higher than among heterosexuals.

Syphilis: Next to AIDS, the Worst of All

Syphilis is another major sexually transmitted disease. Syphilis is a genital ulcerative disease. It usually begins with a simple sore on the penis. If it is diagnosed early and treated with appropriate antibiotics, the sores will usually disappear. If the initial diagnosis is missed, the infection can linger without symptoms and develop into *secondary* syphilis, which is characterized by painful and highly contagious open sores. Congenital syphilis can cause stillbirth, death soon after birth, and physical deformity and neurological complications in children who survive. In adults, untreated syphilis can infect the central nervous system, causing paralysis, insanity, blindness, or death. Untreated syphilis is rare today. But like many other STDs, syphilis facilitates the spread of HIV, increasing transmission of the viruses at least two- to five-fold. The rate of primary and secondary syphilis decreased throughout the 1990s. In 2004, it reached an all-time low. Between 2000 and 2005, a more daunting statistical reality began developing. There was a dramatic (81 percent) increase of infection for primary and secondary syphilis among men, particularly those having unprotected sex with other men.[3] This subgroup of men is primarily responsible for the overall increase in the national syphilis rate increase.

Genital Herpes: Not the Scourge of the Twenty-First Century

Even more commonly seen is genital herpes. As many as sixty million people in America are infected by the virus, and between eighty and ninety million people carry the antibody.[4] Herpes can lie dormant for long periods of time, only to break out in blister-like lesions on the penis, especially during periods of stress, exhaustion, or illness. Symptoms might also include fever, headache, burning while urinating, and discharge. When the blisters appear, the infection is highly contagious. To a healthy male (i.e., not immune deficient), the herpes blisters are virtually harmless, although they can be uncomfortable. They can be treated with topical ointments or oral medication, and they usually clear up completely in five to seven days. Herpes is *not* the scourge of the twenty-first century. It is a minor thorn in the side of a sexually active man—no more virulent than the common herpes blister on the lip (usually called a "cold sore," and people do not panic over that). Although herpes is *not* curable, or even preventable, in almost all instances, it is no more than a transient, though often irritating, annoyance in healthy men and women whose immune systems are intact. Remember, a cold sore on your mouth or penis is perhaps unsightly for a day or two, but it is totally harmless.

I see some men with human papilloma virus (HPV), which can cause warts that look a bit like tiny cauliflowers on the genitals. The warts are not only unsightly (thereby inhibiting the expression of penis power), but the virus is also highly contagious. Most of these lesions are removed with a topical application of a weak, vinegar-like chemical (urologists call it the "pickle wrap"). Stubborn growths might require electrocautery, liquid nitrogen freezing, or laser ablation. Once acquired, HPV can remain invisible and dormant and, similar to herpes, can reappear throughout the life of an infected person. There is mounting evidence that HPV can possibly cause cervical cancer in women. It is incumbent upon any responsible man to be treated promptly and make his partner aware of his condition should he acquire HPV.

AIDS: *The* Scourge of the Twenty-First Century

With respect to penis power, genital infections can definitely cramp your style. Not only can they cause pain or irritation, but no responsible man should engage in sex if it means infecting his partner. Some STDs can cause temporary loss of libido and diminished capacity to obtain an erection. With proper, prompt treatment, these problems are short-lived. The good news is that virtually all of the common sexually transmitted infections, with the notable exception of AIDS, can be completely cured or are self-limited.

Acquired immune deficiency syndrome (AIDS) is a very different story. The virus that causes AIDS, human immunodeficiency virus (HIV), is found in bodily fluids and attacks the cells of the immune system, leaving the body so vulnerable to bacteria, viruses, and parasites that the outcome is almost invariably death. So far there is no known cure for AIDS, but the development of highly effective treatment regimens is prolonging the life of HIV-positive patients far beyond what we were capable of doing even ten years ago.

While the two most susceptible groups remain homosexual men and intravenous drug users, the incidence among heterosexuals is rising. While heterosexuals face a greater statistical risk of dying from drunk driving or not wearing seat belts, do not make the mistake of underestimating the danger of HIV. As Magic Johnson's dramatic announcement in 1991 demonstrated, nobody is above the risk of HIV infection. Despite his robust survival, the infection and deaths of many other celebrity figures since that time has reinforced that this is not the age for casual sex with strangers. Superpotent men who are not in long-term relationships have to adjust to a new reality. When you have sex with someone, you are in a sense sleeping with everyone with whom that person has had sex during the last ten years or more.

As of this writing, the Centers for Disease Control (CDC) in Atlanta recommends that heterosexuals protect themselves by having sexual relations only with low-risk partners. Unfortunately, it is becoming increasingly more difficult to delineate low-risk from high-risk partners as the AIDS epidemic spreads at a frightening speed. HIV-positive infection, once rare in the heterosexual community, has a rate of penetrance that *nearly equals* the spread observed among homosexuals.

According to the Los Angeles Department of Health Services, the overall number of AIDS cases is increasing in *all* racial and ethnic groups. A recent statistical report from the county noted a marked *decrease* in the overall rate of infection among blacks and Hispanics, even though blacks currently account for 50 percent of all newly diagnosed HIV/AIDS cases. The most numerous cases in absolute numbers of infection come from male-to-male sexual contact, across all racial and ethnic lines.[5] However, the lines of AIDS demarcation are increasingly difficult to define. For example, a woman, even though not an intravenous drug user, can nonetheless be infected with the HIV virus from a sexual partner who is an intravenous drug user. She can then, in turn, transmit the virus to her subsequent sexual partners. They, in turn, can pass it on to their partners and so on—less like the domino effect and more like a fission explosion. That is exactly what has happened in Africa and around the world!

As a superpotent man picking a sexual partner, remember that the entire template of that partner's *prior* sexual experience will be permanently tattooed upon you. Those cultures or subcultures that encourage multiple sexual partners (such as young men in big city bathhouses or teenagers on a sexual rampage) greatly facilitate the spread of HIV. The connection between AIDS and anal and oral sex has classically been implicated as the primary route of spread (excluding contaminated needles and blood products). Fellatio by itself *can* transmit HIV. The deadly virus can, in fact, find its way into your bloodstream through any minor break or crack, either in your skin or in the mucous membranes lining any body cavity.

To be informed is to be armed in the war against AIDS. Since there is no cure, extreme caution in both your choice of sexual partners and your sexual menu becomes your only defense. When in doubt, either about a potential partner or a sexual practice, you must simply say no. It is not enough to know that your partner has passed an AIDS test, as the virus can be transmitted before it shows up in a test. In addition, you should heed the usual advice about using condoms or avoiding intercourse. I know condoms may cramp your style (some patients compare it to taking a shower with their socks on). I know sex feels a lot better without them. But your life is at stake. You can love sex even with latex. If you play by the new ground rules, you can still exercise your penis power to your heart's content. You just have to do it with discernment, caution, and care.

Chapter 11

What Women Need to Know

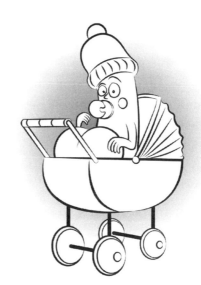

Some say that the way to a man's heart is through his stomach. While that may be true, in my opinion, the way to a man's *soul* is through his penis.

That is the message I want to send to all women. If I had my way, every woman would be a penis expert—a walking encyclopedia of penis knowledge, a veritable wizard at enhancing penis power. My advice to women is to help your man become superpotent. Learn everything you can about the penis: how it works, why it works, when it works, and where it works. Find out what his penis needs, what it likes, what excites it, what makes it "get up and go." Cater to his penis, and it will cater to you. I say this to all women with no regrets because I honestly believe that those women who learn to enhance the penis power of the men in their lives benefit from the happiness that superpotency brings to a relationship.

I say this without hesitation, knowing full well that some women will think it sounds retrograde or sexist. I assure you my message is neither. I am in total support of equality in every aspect of life: at home, at work, and especially in the bedroom. I am an outspoken advocate for women fulfilling themselves in every possible way. I would never suggest that women should become sex slaves, bimbos, or sluts. I am not advocating that women should be subservient or submit to any form of abuse or degradation. What I *am* doing is advising women to make your man's sexual satisfaction a high priority *for your own selfish reasons*. Make *him* happy, and he will make *you* happy. Give *to* him, and you are more likely to get what you want *from* him *quid pro quo*. It is a simple fact of life and a basic principle of human interaction: we do things to please other people because we want them to treat us well. The Golden Rule is never more powerful than when applied to the penis: "Do unto him as you wish he do unto you."

Obviously, the give-and-take nature of sexual relationships works both ways. I spend a great deal of time advising men to learn how to satisfy the women in their lives. With great respect to women, I believe they understand this principle better than men. Women comprehend it instinctively.

Over the years, hundreds of women have taken me aside, whether in my office or at a party, and asked me what they can do to enhance their partner's penis power. They might not use those exact words. They might stammer a little bit. They might beat around the bush and conjure up every euphemism they can think of, but they always want to know the secrets for improving their man's sexuality. This is not, I must add, because they are overcome by selfless generosity, but because they are interested in their own satisfaction. I have never met a woman who did not want a superpotent man because I have never met a woman who did not want to be satisfied herself.

Ladies and Gentlemen: It Begins with Communication

When I get a patient who complains about another doctor, the grievance is invariably "He didn't communicate with me, Doc." Communication, even with doctor-patient interactions, is a fundamental aspect in maintaining a healthy and happy relationship. For this reason, I am sure that marriage counselors and sex therapists hear the same thing all the time from couples who are having relationship problems. It is impossible to overemphasize the importance of communication, especially with regard to sex.

Ladies, if the man in your life does not openly let you know what he likes sexually, then there are essentially three things you can do: forget about it, experiment, or straight out ask him what he likes. I do not recommend the first alternative because any type of sexual ignorance between you and your partner will only have harmful effects on your sex life. The "forget about it" point of view eventually leads to frustration, resentment, and anxiety associated with sex. Learning what turns your partner on and delivering it as best you can is the most effective way to improve his penis power. You can experiment by trying different strategies to see what does and does not work. If your man is not the expressive type, then the answers might not be so obvious. That is why it is important to explore and experiment to your heart's content, which will invariably add to the variety of your experience and help you to learn your partner's tastes. I strongly recommend that you talk to him specifically about *his* needs, his desires, and even his fantasies. By asking him what *he* likes, you will be letting him know that you care about his happiness and that you want to satisfy him in every way you can.

Some men are uncomfortable with candid sex talk. If that is the case, be patient. Get whatever information you can and wait for the next opportunity to get more information. You might also use a book or magazine article as a starting point: "I read that some men like . . ." You can also learn a lot while making love. There is nothing wrong with asking, "Do you like this?" or "Would you like me to . . .?" or "Was that good?" He only has to grunt a response, and you will gather important information about his likes and dislikes.

As I have stated, communication is a two-way street. You want to make sure he understands *your* likes and dislikes because that information will also increase his penis power. You cannot expect him to read your mind, so talk to him openly. Be sure to exercise all of your diplomatic skills. Men have extremely delicate egos, especially when it pertains to their penises. If you want your man to improve his lovemaking abilities, use positive reinforcement as much as possible. Try to avoid saying anything that could be taken as a put-down, especially *while* making love. If you want to correct him or change his behavior, do it delicately and with compassion, as you would with a child. Making him feel self-conscious will probably *diminish* his penis power, even though you are trying to increase it. Be honest and forthright. Focus on what you would *like* him to do, not what he is doing wrong. If you do not like some of his techniques, instead of telling him bluntly, try telling him what you would *rather* he do. In other words, instead of saying, "I cannot stand it when you do that to my breasts," you could say something like, "I think I'd really like it if you did . . . "

Even delicate matters such as early ejaculation can be handled this way. Instead of saying "I think you have a problem" or "Can't you learn to control yourself?" you might use words to the effect of "Making love to you is so wonderful. Wouldn't it be great if we could do it even longer? Let's try to work on it together." The difference is obvious. One form of expression suggests that he is inadequate, while the other says that he is okay, you love him, and you want everything between you to be even better. Even if you think you are joking or innocently pointing out a problem, his fragile penis ego might take it as a put-down. If you say anything that makes him feel defensive, it will surely increase his self-doubt, and you know what self-doubt leads to—performance anxiety and eventually, penis failure.

It is also important for women to try not to come across as overly demanding. Nothing is more intimidating to a man than a woman who makes unrealistic penis demands or issues ultimatums. If you say (or even imply), "Shape up or else!" even a superpotent man might not rise to the occasion. More often than not, a man who gets a message like that will either never be heard from again, or he'll become so nervous that he has a penis power outage.

When your man does something you like, or if he shows any sign of trying to comply with your wishes, give him immediate positive reinforcement. Let him know you like it. Let him know he is on the right track. Let him know you appreciate the effort, even if you have to exaggerate to get that positive message across. The slightest sign of pleasure from you will make your man feel a foot taller. It will reinforce his confidence. That will, in turn, boost his penis power. You might be thinking that this amounts to treating a grown man like a child. Well, in a sense, it is. A man with an erection is more like a child than an adult. Besides, if it ends up making him a superpotent man, what is wrong with a little child psychology?

Women's Top Ten Complaints

In addition to the obvious problems—"He loses his erections at the worst times" and "He ejaculates prematurely"—both of which are discussed at great length elsewhere in this book, I hear several complaints repeatedly from women. What follows is a list of their top ten and a brief discussion of each complaint.

1. "He wants to have sex when I'm not in the mood."

Men typically want sex more often than women, and many of them expect their women to deliver on demand. This is a very sensitive issue because respect and consideration should be the top priority for anyone in an intimate relationship. A smart woman might consider doing everything possible to enable her man to exercise his penis power. Naturally, there are times when it is appropriate to say no; only a Neanderthal would not understand that. By the same token, there are times when it is appropriate to say yes, even if you are not in the mood or would rather be doing something else. In a good relationship, compromise is crucial. This is true for sex, as well as other matters. If he is willing to give in on issues that concern you, why consider it sexist or exploitive if you give in sexually from time to time? This whole issue boils down to a matter of negotiation. If your man is expressing his sexual desire and you are not willing to cater to his needs, then speaking openly about why you are feeling otherwise is the best way to curb his frustration. This is especially important if the reasons for not having sex are emotional or somehow related to issues in your relationship. Discussing all issues openly is the key.

Every couple has to work out their own ground rules. In general, my point of view is that a woman who wants a happy, healthy man will try to be there for him whenever and wherever he wants her. The ultimate beneficiary of your generosity will be you.

2. "Sometimes he turns me down when I want him."

Most men find a sexually aggressive woman a big turnon. They love it when a woman initiates sex, and they love being seduced. It is also true that an overly aggressive woman can threaten a man. Therefore, it is important to find the right balance. Let him know you want him, but do not come on so strong that he feels intimidated.

Of course, some men *hate* it when women initiate sex. Men who are more conservative feel this way for what I believe to be ridiculous and outdated ideological reasons: they feel it is a man's place to "get things rolling." Others simply interpret a woman's assertiveness as demanding. My advice for you is to try every weapon in your arsenal. If he continues to be a reluctant lover, it might be a sign of deeper problems in the relationship.

Of course, his hesitancy might also be due to something completely unrelated to your seductiveness or your relationship. He might be too busy to think about sex or stressed by work. I often get this message from the wives of "movers and shakers." My response is always the same: no man should be too busy to make love to his partner. Women who are in relationships with men like this should try what his business associates do when they want his attention: make an appointment. Tell him you want to set aside a definite time to devote entirely to lovemaking. Rent a hotel room near his office if you must. What a great way to rekindle the romance!

3. "He's so businesslike when we make love!"

It is commonly said that once a man with a hard penis reaches a certain point of arousal, he loses not only his reason but also his sense of humor, his vocal chords, and any semblance of refinement. When a man is sexually charged and ready to go, his animal instincts take over. To a man who is sexually charged, all that matters is ejaculating in a warm hole. Gone is the playfulness, the passion of the ardent lover, the sweet words, the grace, and the charm. He is suddenly a mute, while at the same time he is wild and flailing.

The truth is, if you are looking for a lover with the elegance of Pierce Brosnan and the smoothness of James Bond, you might have to rethink your expectations. If you want a more playful man, one who can laugh and have fun while making love instead of taking it so seriously, then you have a better chance of making some changes in your man. Many men get overly serious because they are nervous about their performance. They are afraid that if they lighten up, they might lose their desire or their erection. You might be able to lead the way to laughter by taking the initiative and making him feel as comfortable as possible. As for whispering in your ear and telling you he loves you, if you do it first and he cannot return the sentiment, have a talk with him *after* you make love. It is hard to teach passion and romance, but a satisfied man might be willing to work on his manners.

On the whole, women often have to accept the fact that some men are *all* business when they are sexually aroused. For these men, sex is the ultimate test of goal-oriented behavior. You have to assess for yourself which of your man's traits you have a chance of changing and which ones you will have to learn to accept.

4. "Sometimes he does things that hurt me."

Sex should always provide mutual pleasure, not pain. I hear two kinds of complaints from women in this regard. The first has to do with clumsy or rough behavior during foreplay: "He bites my nipples like they are cookies," "He rams his fingers in my vagina like a battering pole," or "He rubs my clitoris like he is polishing his car." Men in the throes of sexual passion sometimes lose their sensibilities to lust, and they can become insensitive to their partner's physical and emotional feelings. In addition, some men develop crude and clumsy habits when they first start having sex, and unfortunately, nobody has ever smoothed out those rough spots. A man might simply be uninformed sexually. He might actually think you *like* what he is doing. He may have known women who *did* like it. You absolutely must let him know that he is hurting you. If you can possibly help it, avoid getting angry. Do not let his missteps ruin the experience for you. Tell him gently so he does not take it as criticism or a sign of failure. Hopefully, he will make the appropriate changes. If he continues to ignore your requests and behaves improperly after you talk to him, and if you choose not to end the relationship, then a more serious reprimanding is appropriate. Any woman who finds herself in a relationship that is sexually abusive should either seek counseling or distance herself from that man until he makes serious changes in his behavior.

The other kind of pain that is reported to me occurs during intercourse and includes too much internal friction (which might be solved by a vaginal lubricant), thrusting too hard against the pubic bone, yanking or twisting the body in an awkward manner, and leaning his weight on a tender spot. In each case, you have to help him change his habits. One source of pain, however, is biologically determined: a penis that is too big. As I have already discussed, I have had many more requests to make a husband's penis shorter or thinner than to make it longer or wider. Unfortunately, there is no medical solution to the problem of size. The answer is to adjust the angle of penetration and the depth of insertion until you find a combination that is both satisfying and comfortable. Remember, no rule says a penis has to penetrate to its full length. Communication and experimentation are the best solutions for working out the intricate details of any sexual relationship.

5. "He wants me to do things I find distasteful."

Both partners in a relationship should respect each other's limitations and uphold each other's values. Communicating and establishing personal boundaries is essential for any intimate relationship to be fulfilling for both partners. Unless he's forcing you to do something painful or dangerous, you might want to ask yourself if you are being too prudish.

It comes as no surprise that many women complain that their partners expect them to perform oral sex, which they find abhorrent. If you are one of those women, you should not feel ashamed of your reluctance to take his penis in your mouth. On the other hand, you should examine the source of your resistance—there is nothing inherently dangerous, dirty, or evil about oral sex. Many women find it extremely stimulating, especially if they are madly in love with their partners and enjoy bringing them pleasure.

Perhaps your problem is not so much having a penis in your mouth, but the possibility of swallowing semen. If so, you might have to negotiate with your man. Offer to do it only until he is ready to ejaculate. While many men find it incredibly exciting to climax in their partner's mouths, you might be able to work out a compromise. There is also no rule that says you have to swallow his semen; you can spit it out just as easily. You should also know that, medically speaking, there is no danger in swallowing semen unless it is infected. Semen is not a waste product like urine. Quite the contrary, it is the most vital fluid in the male body. Without it, human life would be extinct. Ingesting semen does not produce negative side effects. It does nauseate some but, in my experience, that is more a psychological than biological reaction.

For the most part, it is simply a matter of taste. Perhaps one day medical science will find ways of altering the flavor of semen, making it more palatable to women who have an aversion to it. Some women have reported that different foods can make semen take on a different flavor or aroma.

If there are other things besides oral sex that your partner is demanding from you that you find distasteful, such as anal sex, uncomfortable or awkward positions, or sex in strange places or at awkward times, then the best solution is to communicate your aversion to his requests. After speaking openly about your feelings, he will hopefully be willing to change of his own accord. If he is unwilling or persists, you may want to seek professional counseling to work through your differences.

6. "My husband is a 'wham-bam thank-you ma'am' kind of guy, and all he knows is the missionary position."

The simple solution to these issues is to educate him! In a gentle way, let him know that you enjoy being intimate with him so much that you would like to savor the experience by slowing down and making each moment last. You can even ask him, "What's the rush?" Teach him that an extra few minutes of loving foreplay or passionate intercourse will bring *both* of you heightened pleasure.

Keep in mind that sometimes every man acts as if he is in a race to ejaculate. Sometimes men are simply overcome by a physical need, and their instincts take over, even if their minds are screaming, "Slow down!" If such occurrences are the *exception*, and not the rule, you should be able to tolerate it from time to time, even if it means that only one of you leaves the bed satisfied. This does not mean you should tolerate crude or thoughtless behavior. If the "quickie" is the norm all of the time, then communicating your frustration by asking him to be more considerate of your needs and modify his in-bed behavior can be the best way to initiate change.

As for trying new things, if your man has a limited imagination, then lend him yours. Make explicit suggestions. If that does not work, try nonverbal communication—take the bull by the horns and maneuver creatively until you make him an offer he cannot refuse.

7. "My lover does not want me to touch his penis."

This is not a common problem. When it does happen, it can be both difficult and saddening. For a woman who wants to express her affection by caressing her loved one, it can be terribly unpleasant to have her hand pushed aside or be told "No!" It occurs most often in new relationships and usually stems from one of two things: the man is afraid of premature ejaculation or he has an abnormal, deep-rooted fear of being touched. The first scenario is easier to deal with and usually improves as soon as the man feels secure in his performance. The second scenario is more intractable and takes patience to overcome. I recommend gradual steps to make him comfortable with the idea of being fondled. The longest journey begins with the first step. Instead of *grabbing* his penis, start by stroking it with one finger for a short amount of time or rubbing it with your thigh or arm, and work your way gradually to normal manual stimulation. Treat his reluctant penis with gentle kid gloves until his fears dissipate.

8. "Sometimes he annoys me so much I cannot bring myself to have sex with him, even though I'm feeling sexual."

Every couple has their run of conflicts and problems, and everyone has their own set of pet peeves that sometimes drive them crazy. The secret to making an intimate relationship last is to find a way to ignore the things you cannot change. To be blunt, get over it—even if it is for no other reason than to satisfy yourself. If there is a deep and serious rift in the relationship, by all means work it out, either privately or with a counselor. If your relationship is getting thrown off track by the normal, run-of-the-mill irritations that affect every relationship, then do yourself a favor: do not let that get in the way of sex. If you do, not only will both of you end up frustrated, but you will be neglecting the best solution to your problem. I am reminded of Sutton's Law. When the infamous bank robber Willie Sutton was asked why he robbed banks, he replied, "Because that's where the money is." Danoff's Law states: "Satisfy your man's penis because that's where his soul is." After a good roll in the hay, you will have worked off that frustration, you will feel relaxed, and your man will be much more amenable to sympathizing with your grievances and working toward a resolution.

9. "When my husband has a few drinks, all he wants to do is have sex, but I don't like him in that condition."

If your man needs a little booze to lower his inhibitions or to free his mind of troubles, it is not necessarily a bad thing. Unfortunately, many women have told me that too much alcohol can turn an amorous man into a clumsy, insensitive brute. It can also keep his penis from reaching the launching pad. Like so many other problems, this one requires diplomacy. You should tell him why you prefer to make love when he *has not* been drinking. If you want to be understood, make sure you have the conversation with him when he is sober. If, on the other hand, your partner has a serious drinking or drug problem, one that is a threat to his own health and is causing problems in your relationship and love life, then you should recommend he seek professional treatment immediately. You should do whatever it takes to help him overcome his destructive dependence.

10. "I'm a single mother. How can I educate my son about penis power?"

The most important thing you can do as a single parent is to provide your son with unconditional love and let him know at every possible opportunity that he's worthy of his own self-respect. If you raise a healthy, self-assured son, the chances are he will feel secure in his penis image. As to the details of a young man's penis education, you can provide him with facts as easily as a man can, but you cannot speak from experience and you cannot be a role model. If you have a male relative or close male friend whom you and your son trust, someone who can take your son under his wing and teach him about his body and his sexuality, then you can compensate to some degree for the absence of a father. If the surrogate is a man of true superpotency, his presence might serve your son's penis education better than a real father who is not around.

Penis-Oriented Women Have More Fun

Hopefully, the preceding section has answered some of the tougher questions about men, the issues surrounding the penis, and some female queries about male sexuality. I encourage women who may still have unanswered questions to do everything in their power to become as well educated as possible in all matters pertaining to the penis. A woman who is penis oriented is not only able to manage a relationship better but is also empowered to create her own happiness. My observations have led me to conclude that penis-oriented women not only have more fun, they also have better marriages, more faithful husbands, happier homes, and greater personal fulfillment in all aspects of their lives. I assure you that if women would spend as much time attending to their man's penis as they devote to their hair, makeup, and clothing, they would get more of what they want and have a far more satisfying relationship. If you accept the premise, as I do, that men are dominated to a large degree by the imperatives of their penises, and if you believe that each partner has the mutual responsibility to satisfy the other's needs, then it follows that you will hold up your end of the bargain by making his penis one of your top priorities.

Being penis oriented does *not* imply a belittlement of female sexuality. It does not make you less of a feminist or less than an equal to the men in your life. It does not require that you sacrifice your intelligence or your self-respect. It simply means learning to understand and accommodate a man's penis needs by approaching that task with all of the pride and skill that you would bring to any other endeavor. I assure you that, based on all of my clinical experience, if you take the steps to become informed, you and your man will reap rewards you have only dreamed about.

Chapter 12

Penis FAQs

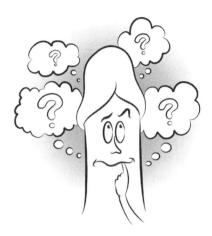

Because the average person knows so little about the area in which I specialize, I spend a great deal of time responding to all types of questions from patients, friends, and sometimes even strangers. In this chapter, I will address some of the questions that I am frequently asked that have not yet been fully covered elsewhere in this book.

Q: Do women prefer certain kinds of penises to others?

A: This is probably the single most significant penis question on the minds of the men with whom I have talked over the years. In my many years of urologic practice, I have had thousands of conversations with women about the most intimate details of their sex lives. They have told me things they have related to no other person, including their most esoteric sexual practices and wildest fantasies. For the most part, women do not ever seriously express to me a strong preference for one kind of penis over another. Believe me, I have asked! However, it cannot be denied that when it comes to penises, some women do have a definite preference as to size or shape. But the overwhelming majority of women I have interviewed have confessed that length, width, appearance, and complexion are all factors that do not seem to matter in a long-term relationship, even to the women who describe in detail the specific kinds of chests, legs, and behinds that excite them in their mates.

The only real complaints I have heard are regarding what we call a micropenis. This is an abnormally small penis. The true micropenis is extremely rare. It is at the low end of the bell-shaped curve. Ultimately, with the exception of those men who lie outside the middle of the curve, I stand by the belief that men can be as "big" as they think they are. In reality, penis size is not as significant as most men believe it to be because the penis is not the only body part that can be used to stimulate and satisfy a partner. Whether or not penis size is an issue for you as a man or an issue within a sexual relationship, as a superpotent man, you must learn to use your hands, lips, tongue, or any other device that can aid in stimulating your partner.

For the majority, when it comes to the penis, what partners care about most is *hardness* and *responsiveness*; some also mention cleanliness. The penis is a functional organ, not necessarily an aesthetic object. For this reason, some women may require a larger functioning penis to stimulate them to orgasm. In most cases, this is simply an anatomical fact (a taller or larger woman will invariably have more body fat, creating a greater distance over which an erect penis must traverse, or a larger vagina that requires a larger penis for stimulation). It is important for the two partners to *communicate* their physical needs and personal desires. Experimenting with different positions and alternative or additional methods of stimulation can help satisfy both partners and go a long way toward maintaining a strong emotional and sexual relationship.

Some women and some homosexual men have a preconditioned attraction to a large penis as a sign of masculinity. They make a psychological association between large penises and their own satisfaction. This association is not only erroneous but it is also an unhealthy way of gauging the potential of a man. It is important for men and women to recognize that sexual satisfaction is not limited to the penis, and especially not to its size or shape.

As in all things, knowledge is power, and I cannot stress enough how much the sexual power of a man can be elevated when he simply learns how to cater to the specific and unique needs of his partner. Ultimately, the penis, regardless of its size, is one of many sexual tools that men have at their disposal. The more you learn how to use your entire body to stimulate your partner, the less important one part of the body becomes.

Q: Is there a legitimate way to make my penis any larger?

A: The answer is unequivocally no! Many men come to me with questions about a variety of "enlarging" procedures known collectively as phalloplasty. Surgeons have and are using a number of techniques, including skin grafts (known as dermal matrix grafts), in an attempt to increase the girth of the penis. These procedures, as well as a lengthening technique that increases penis length by severing the suspensory ligaments, are falsely represented as legitimate ways to increase the size of the penis. I cannot emphasize to my patients enough that phalloplasty and lengthening procedures are both inventions of hucksters, charlatans, and fakes. Not only are they ineffective, they are also highly risky. The idea that men need to have huge penises is a cultural myth perpetuated more by men than by women. There is hardly a man alive who does not dream of a bigger penis. Be assured there is no medically or surgically effective way of doing this safely at the present time. To believe otherwise is to subject your penis to gross disfigurement.

Q: If I have sex a lot, can I damage my penis?

A: The chances of injuring your penis are miniscule, no matter how vigorously you exercise it. Nature has designed your penis to be tough, resilient, and durable. It can take much more of a thrashing than most other appendages. Try twisting your ear or bending a finger the way you can bend your penis. It can even stand getting whacked around more than most organs, although I suggest that you take my word on that and not experiment on your own.

With the exception of whales, no mammals have bones in their penises, although some mammals have an *os*, which is simply a bone-like appendage made up of rigid connective tissue. In human males, there is no bone in the penis, and so nothing to fracture. Nor are there ligaments, joints, or muscles to strain or tear. Surrounding the corpora cavernosa (the chamber in the shaft of the penis that fills with blood) is a fibrous tunica, tissue so tough that I have to apply extreme pressure just to incise it when performing surgery. When the penis is erect and the corpora is filled with blood, it is possible that a sharp blow or trauma can rupture this fibrous sheath (tunica). Such incidents are extremely rare and are mistakenly called a "fractured penis." This is a misnomer. It is also possible to rupture the surface capillaries of the penis, causing discoloration and bruising. This is also unusual, especially in the context of even vigorous sexual activity.

If you still have doubts, you should look to your own experience for validation: how many men have you known who have injured their penises compared to those who have damaged their hands, arms, feet, or legs? If you can recall any man complaining of a penis injury, chances are it had to do with the *skin*. The skin is the most vulnerable part of the penis. It can suffer abrasions, cuts, and bruises, but these occur more often from accidents. Getting your penis stuck in a zipper is the most common cause, rather than through ordinary sexual activity. The most frequent sex-related injury is skin irritation caused by excessive friction. This kind of irritation keeps more men from having sex than any other injury and is why one of my colleagues believes that "lubricants have saved more marriages than Dear Abby." It is also possible to bruise the glans (the head of the penis) by thrusting against a woman's pubic bone or other hard body part. Again, traumatic injuries are more often caused by something *other* than ordinary sex.

Unfortunately, most of the penis injuries I see in my office and in the emergency room are self-inflicted. You would not believe the number of objects I have removed from penises throughout my career—not just rings and clips that perforate the skin, but long, thin items inserted into the urethra, including pencils, pens, pins, wires, and especially swizzle sticks (drink mixers).

The bottom line is, you only have one penis, so use it, don't abuse it!

Q: If I use my penis a lot sexually, will it become weaker or "burn out" as I get older?

A: There is no predetermined number of orgasms, no quota of erections or ejaculations, and no upper limit that can be exceeded. Your seminal vesicles will not dry up if you ejaculate too much. Your penis will not become flaccid if you have sex a thousand times. Fortunately, nature has not rationed sexuality. You may get fatigued from having a lot of sex, just as you would from *any* physical activity. Your body is smart: if you get too fatigued, you lose your sexual desire. Get some rest, and your libido will promptly return. If you use your penis frequently and vigorously, it will invigorate the rest of your body and keep your spirit young and vibrant. Penis *under-use* is a much bigger problem than *overuse*.

Q: I have a history of heart disease. Do I have to limit my sexual practices?

A: Every heart patient should be advised according to his specific condition and consult with his cardiologist prior to vigorous activity of any kind, including sex. However, I must dispel the myth that having sex is damaging to the heart. In the past, men who survived heart attacks were often told not to have sex. They were also told not to exercise and to retire from physically demanding work. We now know that, within appropriate limits, exercise is good for heart patients. In that respect, sex is no different. It is not only a terrific form of exercise, but it is also unsurpassed in lifting the spirit of a man who has suffered the trauma of a heart attack. Men with cardiac disorders often get depressed. They feel old, and their performance anxiety suffers. These psychological factors can impede their penis power. There is no better antidote for such masculine malaise than having sex.

I must, however, issue an important caveat. If you have a history of heart disease, you should not be overdoing *anything*, including sex. As with any form of exercise, if you get chest pain while having sex, stop immediately and see your cardiologist as soon as possible. One problem I frequently see in older men with cardiovascular problems is that they sometimes experience retarded ejaculation, meaning a delayed ejaculation. Because it takes them longer to reach climax, these men get caught up in a frenzy of exertion, aiming for the elusive orgasm. This is like pushing the limits of your endurance to reach the finish line ahead of your opponent. It is fine for a well-conditioned man, but to someone with cardiovascular disease, it can be extremely dangerous. If you are an older man and have experienced cardiovascular problems, take your time during sex. Do not try to overdo it. If you do not recognize your limits and adjust your practices accordingly, dire consequences can ensue.

One other caution: if you suffer from coronary artery disease and have occasional exertion-related chest pain (angina) and you treat the pain with nitroglycerin, you should *never* take any of the oral medications for erectile dysfunction (Viagra, Levitra or Cialis). Each of these PDE-5 inhibitors is a potent vasodilator, and in combination with nitroglycerin (also a potent vasodilator), the two drugs can cause a fatal drop in blood pressure.

In conclusion, it is important to make intelligent decisions as you age. Do not be afraid to express yourself sexually as your body begins to change, but do not be a hero either. Make it a point to discuss your sex life with your cardiologist as candidly as you would your exercise routine.

Q: Is it possible to become addicted to sex?

A: From a medical standpoint, the answer is no. Our criterion for addiction is based on the presence of physiological symptoms of *withdrawal*. When an addict is deprived of that to which he is addicted, he will suffer predictable biochemical consequences (as with alcohol, nicotine, or narcotics). Being deprived of sex does not feel good, and different men will suffer to a lesser or greater extent. However, that does not constitute addiction any more than suffering over a lack of food makes you a food addict or feeling restless because you have not worked out makes you an exercise junkie. Like food and exercise, sex is nonaddictive.

More accurately, men can become *compulsive* about or *obsessed* with sex. In extreme cases, this can impact negatively on other aspects of life. Sexual obsession is not *caused* by too much sexual activity. It is not like taking heroine or cocaine; you do not become addicted or dependent by having frequent sex. Rather, destructive sexual obsession is usually a function of deep-rooted psychological problems and not a matter of addiction. Men with that condition should seek consultation with a qualified psychotherapist.

Q: If I take testosterone, will I become a better lover?

A: As discussed in chapter 9, unless your testosterone level is abnormally low to begin with, taking supplementary testosterone by injection or topical application (when your serum testosterone level is within the normal range) will not change your ability to get or keep an erection. It will not improve your sexual capacity in any way. In fact, taking excessive amounts of testosterone can be physically detrimental. If you do take excess testosterone, the result will be "tiny testes." Your urologist will diagnose testicular atrophy, a condition not uncommon in athletes, and particularly in bodybuilders who use anabolic steroids. What testosterone *might* do is increase your level of sexual desire, but it will not add a thing to your performance. (See chapter 9 "As Old as You Feel: The Life

Story of the Penis," for more information on the subject of testosterone replacement therapy, or TRT.)

Q: My friends seem to be more interested in sex than I am. Is there something wrong with me?

A: Levels of desire can vary widely among men. One study of college students had the subjects press a counter every time they had a sexual thought or fantasy. Some students clicked more than three hundred times a day, while others reported they rarely had a sexual thought. Who is to say what is normal and what is not? What's important is that you are personally able to satisfy whatever level of sexual desire you have. If you find you have a paucity of interest in pursuing sexual encounters or you are too afraid or too busy to engage in romance, take the time to examine the reasons. You may be avoiding intimate relationships; you may have an aversion to sex. If you feel intimidated by sex because of bad experiences in the past, follow the advice I have outlined throughout this book. Think positively. Move forward. Do not dwell on past experiences if they were less than satisfactory.

Q: I am thinking of having a vasectomy. Will it affect my penis power?

A: Vasectomy is a safe, effective method of birth control for men who no longer wish to have children. The procedure involves interrupting the continuity of the vas deferens, the tube that carries sperm from the testicles, where sperm is made, to the seminal vesicles, where sperm is stored until ejaculation. Basically, vasectomy stops only the *passage* of sperm, so that none of it is included in the semen you ejaculate. The procedure itself is performed in less than ten minutes in my office under a local anesthesia through a tiny nick in the scrotal skin (the "no scalpel" technique). The postoperative discomfort is minimal and rarely requires analgesics.

As for penis power, *absolutely no change occurs after a vasectomy.* There is no reduction in sensation, no lowering of desire, no less circulating testosterone, no loss of ability to get or keep an erection, and no less satisfaction when having an orgasm. The only difference after a vasectomy is that you release no sperm. Sperm comprises a miniscule portion of the seminal fluid to begin with, so there is no reduction in the volume of semen that is ejaculated.

For many men, a vasectomy has the potential to *increase* penis power because they are no longer inhibited by concerns about pregnancy. Long-time partners often feel more spontaneous. They do not have to interrupt lovemaking to deal with diaphragms or condoms, and they often feel heightened sensation during intercourse because there is no latex between the penis and the vagina.

Some vasectomy patients change their minds about having children and request a reversal. This procedure, called a vasovasostomy, involves reconnecting the vas deferens. This is a more difficult procedure than the original vasectomy. However, this operation has a high rate of success, and most patients are able to conceive children afterward. Just as with a vasectomy, the reversal does not diminish penis power. In fact, there is a potential bonus: after a vasovasostomy, a couple is now making love with the express purpose of conceiving a child. Lovemaking is often more romantic than ever. The typical vasovasostomy patient I see is reversing a vasectomy he obtained when he and his first wife decided not to have any more children. Now he is remarried, usually to a younger woman. The new wife wants to have a family with him—a terrific turnon for a middle-aged man. For a man fitting this profile, I encourage vasovasostomy. It is a safe and effective procedure. Just for the record, the above example is not intended in any way to encourage men to seek divorce, but rather is a reflection of the demographic realities of what I have observed in my clinical practice.

Q: Are there any other alternatives for male birth control?

A: Unfortunately, no other effective and practical alternatives for male birth control exist at this point other than abstinence, a vasectomy, the use of condoms or other prophylactics, or withdrawal. I would predict that with the rapid rate of advances we have seen in medical science, men will soon be able to simply take a pill to control the release of sperm, just as some women take a pill to control the release of their eggs.

Q: I heard that a "cock ring" would help me last longer before ejaculating. Do you recommend the use of such a device?

A: No. In the hope of prolonging intercourse, some men place metallic or elastic constriction rings around the base of their penises after an erection is achieved. Theoretically, the ring impedes the venous outflow, so the blood trapped within the penis shaft cannot escape and the penis stays erect longer. It sounds good in principle, but it can be dangerous. If blood flow is restricted unnaturally—a definite risk with use of the ring—there is a danger of blood sludging or clotting or even rupture of the delicate sinusoids of the penis. When blood is trapped in the penis and cannot escape, a persistent and painful erection can form. This is known as priapism, an uncommon side effect of using a cock ring or similar device. The damage can sometimes be irreversible, making erections in the future more difficult to achieve.

Not long ago, I was called to the emergency room at four in the morning. A man about twenty-four years old who was high on some drug had a thick brass ring circling the base of his penis. It was so tight that it was eroding the skin. When I examined his penis, the arterial blood continued to flow *into* his penis, but the venous *out* flow was shut off, so the penis was grotesquely engorged. I told him we had to give him anesthesia and "saw off" the ring. I left the room to make preparations. When I returned, the patient was gone. He panicked at the thought of someone wielding a saw so close to his penis. He ran from the hospital in panic. I do not know what happened to him, but I do know that, if you want to delay ejaculation, you are better off trying some of the techniques described in chapters 7 and 15.

Q: Ever since my wife gave birth, I do not feel like having sex. What is happening?

A: It is sad to say, but surveys indicate that this is common. One theory holds that postnatal changes in a woman's body might make her less attractive to her husband. For example, some women develop stretch marks on the lower abdomen or varicose veins in the legs, while others might find that their breasts have become less firm. Another finding suggests that the demands of parenting can wear down a mother and exhaust a father. In my mind, the main reason is this: after giving birth, the wife's attention shifts dramatically from her mate to her child. Now that the child consumes her, the bulk of her affection and love are aimed at the baby.

For many women, giving birth brings a stronger sense of fulfillment than any other activity in their lives. It is normal and natural for a mother's energy to be focused on her baby. Unfortunately, even men who share that sense of parental satisfaction and appreciate their wives' commitment to the child might, on some unconscious level, feel rejected. They are suddenly in second place. Such postpartum changes are predictable. They require psychological adjustments and modifications in the timing and circumstances of lovemaking. It is crucial that the superpotent man understand the dynamics at work when a new child is brought into the equation. It is just as important not to interpret his wife's behavior as a form of rejection.

Q: I want sex a lot more than my partner does. What can I do about that?

A: About one-third of the couples seeking marital or relationship help do so because of a marked discrepancy in the desire level of each partner. It is a common problem reflected in the old joke: what do you call foreplay in a marriage? Answer: begging.

No man likes to be rejected, even if he is secure in his partner's love and knows he is adored. No man likes to beg for sex. It is a fact of life that, on average, men have higher levels of desire than women, and they find themselves in the mood for sex more often than women. Unfortunately, the problem can get worse if you suppress your sexual frustration. You run the risk of becoming hostile and resentful, usually letting those feelings out in ways that may have nothing to do with the real issue. You might stop initiating sex altogether rather than face the possibility of rejection. You might begin to shy away from all displays of affection. And, of course, you might be tempted to look elsewhere for sex.

I believe that a superpotent man should do everything in his power to fulfill his sexual needs. Naturally, every man's ideal is to have his partner respond with enthusiasm each and every time he wants to have sex. In reality, coaxing, cajoling, and all forms of seduction might have to be employed, and even some subtle form of bribery (jewelers and florists can attest to that). No one should be reduced to actual begging, although I have a surprisingly large number of patients who are not above pleading. When approached with a sense of humor, even that may be justified. Superpotent men are pragmatic: they do whatever it takes to get the job done.

The best approach is *honest communication*. You must break the silence barrier. Talk openly and candidly about your needs and about the discrepancies in your desire levels. Educate your partner. She might not realize how frustrated you feel. She might not understand how demeaning it is to be told no. She might not understand the importance of sex in your overall happiness. You can never know unless you talk to her—she might be perfectly willing to accommodate you and change her behavior so that you can express yourself sexually. You must also be prepared to listen to her point of view, understand her needs, and negotiate an agreement that can make you both happy. You might have to make some changes yourself, like having sex at different times or initiating it in new ways. If two people care enough about satisfying each other's needs, they can usually overcome the complications that are caused by a difference in levels of desire. If your efforts fail, then it may be time to see a counselor.

Q: Why do I seem to have more penis power in the summer?

A: When it comes to superpotency, hot is better than cold. That is why most couples honeymoon in Hawaii and not the Klondike. It is not only the seductive ambience of tropical flowers, scented air, and hula dancers but also the physical effects of the climate. Have you noticed what happens to your scrotum when you plunge into a cold pool? The skin contracts drastically, the scrotal sac shrinks to the size of a peanut, and the testicles retract into the inguinal canal. Cold also causes vasoconstriction, or narrowing of the blood vessels. None of these conditions is conducive to penis power.

So why all the partying among ski bums and bunnies in frigid ski resorts? After an invigorating day on the slopes, it feels downright tropical by the fireplace, in the hot tub, or under a thick down comforter.

Q: My orgasms are not as explosive as they used to be, and I do not release as much semen. Is something wrong?

A: This is a very common question. Invariably, the men asking it are in their forties (if they are older, they have usually been carrying the question around for a while). As men age, their bodies produce less seminal fluid, so the volume of their ejaculate decreases. This is normal and natural, and every man should expect this change as he ages. The volumetric rule in urology states that ejaculatory volume (semen) is inversely proportional to advancing age. In laymen's terms, this means that the older men get, the less ejaculatory volume they have. This rule also applies to the frequency of intercourse (the older one gets and the more frequent one has intercourse, the smaller the ejaculatory volume becomes). Semen volume is inversely proportional to frequency. Another aspect that is affected by age is the refractory period, the time it takes for the penis to restore itself after ejaculation. The refractory period changes proportionally with age: the older men get, the longer the refractory period becomes. Although this may sound daunting to those young men for whom age is still not a factor in their sex lives, I assure you that the feeling of pleasure and satisfaction you get from an orgasm has nothing to do with the *volume* of your ejaculate.

Why do your orgasms feel less intense? You still enjoy your favorite food, but eating it the hundredth time does not compare to the intensity of previous meals. You still enjoy a good ball game or concert, but the thrill is not quite the same as when you were younger. The more substantive reason for diminished intensity can be found in the complex associations created by your mind. I have had men come in with big grins on their faces, saying that their orgasms have become much more intense ever since they met their new lover. Believe me, the reflex of ejaculation has not changed. The difference is completely in their minds and hearts, where orgasms really take place.

Q: Is there any way to make my orgasms last longer?

A: This is one area where men are jealous of women. I call it "Venus envy." For whatever reason, nature designed humans so that women can have prolonged wavelike orgasms while men can have brief and thunderous orgasms, five to seven seconds in duration. Wouldn't it be great, men dream, if we could make that ecstatic sensation last a full minute? Five minutes? An hour? So far, no one has come up with a way to do that. We have found ways to *delay* orgasm, but not to *prolong* it. (I am told that the Indian tradition of tantric yoga teaches esoteric techniques for extending sexual ecstasy, but I cannot vouch for this as a medical doctor.)

I will go out on a limb and predict that we will find a way to prolong male orgasm somehow, someday. With sex being studied by more scientists than ever before, I feel safe in predicting that researchers will eventually accomplish what most individual men have been unable to do on their own. When that day comes, it will be a great one for men.

Q: Do superpotent men masturbate?

A: There is nothing wrong with masturbation. It is normal. Masturbation should not elicit any form of shame or embarrassment.

However, I want to emphasize that it should be the last resort for the superpotent man. Naturally, every man is alone at times, without an acceptable partner available to relieve his sexual tension. Under such circumstances, masturbation is certainly better than no sexual activity at all. To those men who cannot go through a day without servicing themselves or who are obsessed with watching pornography (especially in today's world of cyberspace and cybersex), I believe they need to re-examine their view of sex. Not only does pornography present a completely unrealistic view of sex in general, but it also has the potential to instill unhealthy habits that can result in serious consequences for future intimate relationships. In short, masturbation will do in a pinch, but it is no substitute for the real thing. Given its negative connotations, too much masturbation can increase levels of self-doubt. One cannot help feeling a bit inadequate if he has to resort to mono when he would rather perform in stereo.

Mutual masturbation is another matter entirely. Couples who know how to use their hands and fingers with the artistry of violinists can fill a bedroom with fantastically erotic music. So it is fine to let your hands do the talking, but it is a whole lot better if the conversation is between two people.

Q: Does circumcision affect penis power?

A: There are no scientifically controlled experiments regarding the sexual performance of circumcised versus uncircumcised men. Based upon my clinical experience, there is no difference. Some people assume that the *circumcised* man has greater sensitivity because he has no foreskin covering the glans. Others believe that the *uncircumcised* man has greater sensitivity because he has a foreskin. Neither theory is true. The fact is that the foreskin retracts when an uncircumcised man has an erection, so in the aroused state, the penises are virtually the same.

Q: Is it wise to circumcise a newborn?

A: My opinion as a urologist is yes. Uncircumcised men have a vastly greater chance of getting penile cancer. In fact, cancer of the penis, which is rare in any case, is virtually unheard of among circumcised men. Recent studies of AIDS prevention in Africa suggest that male circumcision can reduce the chance of HIV in men and perhaps in women. The validity of this is still being tested, but the research shows that the cells on the underside of the foreskin are prime targets for the virus; tears and abrasions in the foreskin serve as an easy port of entry for the retrovirus. Other studies have estimated that circumcised men have a 44 percent lower risk for HIV infection.[1] Although this research is still evolving, it is fair to conclude that circumcision for men should be promoted at least with regard to HIV prevention.

There is also the matter of cleanliness. If an uncircumcised man does not regularly retract the foreskin and wash underneath it, the natural secretions from the skin can produce a smelly, cheesy substance known as smegma. Lack of cleanliness can lead to irritation, pain, and even infection. Many women complain about the odor that results from failing to wash frequently and thoroughly under the foreskin. Generally speaking, circumcision remains a healthier choice, but it has no effect on penis power. I do not recommend it in my adult uncircumcised patients unless a medical problem warrants it such as persistent irritation, infection, rash, or the inability to retract the foreskin for cleaning. Another legitimate reason for circumcision is if a man's sexual partner *requests* that he have one as a matter of personal preference. In any case, an adult circumcision is a quick, simple, and safe procedure when performed by an experienced and qualified urologist.

Q: My doctor says I must have surgery for prostate cancer. I am afraid I will become impotent. Is there any alternative?

A: Let me tell you the story of a patient named Morton. He was a widower in his sixties. He had recently married a woman in her forties. She had the perfect combination of beauty and brains: a former showgirl, who became a lawyer. Morton was having the time of his life with his new bride. It was as if he had discovered the fountain of youth. Then we found a malignant tumor in his prostate. Given his age and the nature and extent of his cancer, the treatment with the greatest likelihood of cure was the surgical removal of his prostate. I told Morton the truth, namely that we could be reasonably certain of curing his cancer but, in spite of employing the robotic nerve-sparing technique, we could not guarantee 100 percent that his ability to get satisfactory erections would be preserved. It was a choice between risking the spread of cancer and potentially risking partial loss of his potency.

Morton was so terrified at the thought of possibly losing perhaps 10 percent of the firmness of his erection that he insisted on an alternative treatment. I recommended the most advanced nerve-sparing surgical procedure available for removing the cancer, which uses the da Vinci laparoscopic robot. There would be no unsightly scar, and the magnification afforded by this technique would allow the most meticulous preservation of the nerves of potency available (see chapter 5, "Prostatic and Other Urologic Diseases," for more details on laparoscopic procedures). Instead of following my recommendation, Morton opted for a far less effective treatment because it promised less potential for loss of penis power. I pleaded with Morton to follow my advice. He declined.

Several years later, I learned that Morton was dying of metastatic prostate cancer. The disease that had started in his prostate was now widely disseminated. Morton was a brilliant and successful businessman with a reputation for making smart decisions. He literally sacrificed his life by thinking with his penis instead of his brain, by trading optimal cancer treatment for a transitory hard penis.

If you are faced with a decision like Morton's, pay attention to your urologist. As medical doctors, we have vast clinical experience and years of training that enable us to sort out all of the variables.

Have your urologist explain exactly what your condition is and what the benefits and risks are with *each* of the alternative treatment methods that are applicable in your particular case. These options might include advanced, focally beamed radiation therapy (IMRT), Brachytherapy (radioactive seeds), cryotherapy (freezing), "watchful waiting," nerve-sparing robotic surgery, or some combination of these procedures. After speaking with your urologist, if you are still unsure about which treatment option suits you best for your age, general medical condition, and the grade and stage of your cancer, get a second opinion, or even a third and fourth if necessary.

Do not hold your life hostage to sex. If those vital nerves must be compromised in surgery to ensure complete ablation of the cancer, you can still be helped with any postoperative erectile dysfunction by utilizing the "the pills" (e.g., Viagra, Cialis, Levitra), a prosthetic penile implant, or an injectable medication. As a surgeon, my first obligation is to cure your cancer. I will do my best to preserve your penis power, but not at the risk of shortening your life. I would hope that other urologists share the same philosophy. (See chapters 5 and 6 for a detailed discussion on the subject of prostate cancer and erectile dysfunction.)

Q: As a father, what can I do to help my son grow up to be a superpotent man?

A: You are your son's primary penis role model. The smallest message from you—a nod, a grunt, a shrug, a casual remark—gets carved into his memory deeper and more permanently than anything he picks up in a sex education class or on the schoolyard. Set a good, responsible example with a *superpotent* attitude. A father who keeps his genitals under cover all the time, never mentions the word *penis*, or avoids his son's questions about sexuality will raise a self-conscious and probably self-doubting son. If you are open and honest and demonstrate penis pride, your son will absorb the right education by example without your having to do much about it.

You can reinforce your example by being candid and up-front about penis matters without making too big a deal about it. Treat the penis as a fact of life, not as something dirty to be hidden behind a zipper or something of great mystery that cannot be spoken about in public. Make sure you are his main source of information—which means it is a top priority for you to be as educated as possible about penis issues. Boys are extremely curious about their penises. If they suppress their curiosity because their parents evade the topic, they will come of age in ignorance or get their penis education the wrong way—from their peers. Do not pull punches, hide behind cute euphemisms, or limit the discussion of these issues to brief moments or offhand comments. It is important to be frank with your son, just as it is important to be casual and lighthearted.

Let me give you an example. When my son turned seven, he asked me, "When will my penis be as big as yours?" I said, "Put your hand in mine. When your fingers are as long as mine, which they definitely will be, then your penis will be as big as my penis." I knew perfectly well that the penis is a special body part (my son would not have bothered asking when his hands or feet would be as big as mine). I treated it as a simple fact of life, no different from fingers or toes. Naturally, the mere fact that a son can ask that question suggests that he grew up in an atmosphere of openness and had occasion to be naked with his father.

As your son grows, make sure he understands penis matters on a level commensurate with his age. Let him know you are there for him and that you have answers should he have penis questions. When boys go through puberty and adolescence, *all* of them wonder if their organ is normal. Let your son know that his penis is perfectly fine, and help build and reinforce his self-confidence by describing the unique and special qualities of the penis: that it is a pleasure-giving appendage that should be appreciated, respected, and used wisely.

Let me give you another simple example from my own life. When I was a teenager, I was very self-conscious about being shorter than many girls at school. I once came home from a party feeling awful. I told my father, "I am really popular, I'm a good dancer, but half the girls are taller than me, and I'm embarrassed to dance with them." My father responded with a big smile that let me know I was okay. Then he said, "You know, son, all girls are the same size lying down."

It was a simple man-to-man moment, but it had a big impact on me. In a subtle way, it instilled in me the confidence to approach *any* girl. (Later on, by the way, I learned that my father was somewhat right anatomically: there is relatively little size difference among most people if you measure from the pubic bone to the neck; it is mainly the length of the legs that creates height differences. When you are horizontal for sexual purposes, height becomes irrelevant, except in extreme cases.)

One caveat is worth mentioning regarding educating your son: sexual candor does not entail prying into your child's life. Teenagers need privacy. If you are *too* meddlesome and *too* up-front, you can intimidate your child. Unnecessary pressure has no place in your relationship with your son. Some fathers think they are instilling positive sexual attitudes by sharing sexy books or movies or alluding to their own exploits. Do not defeat your purpose by creating standards that make your child apprehensive and uncertain. Your son should get the message that he and his penis are okay just the way they are.

Give him that message in every possible way. Superpotency is a matter of penis attitude, and penis attitude is a direct reflection of self-image. Do everything in your power to raise your child to have healthy self-esteem. Let him know that he is loved unconditionally and appreciated for who he is without regard to his performance in school or on the playing field. Teach your child to judge himself by his own standards, not by yours or anyone else's.

Q: What can I do to prevent medical problems in my sexual organs?

A: Unfortunately, the average physician sadly neglects to examine male genitals. Most physical exams, other than those done by urologists, do not even include a cursory examination of the area, perhaps because doctors find it embarrassing or distasteful to touch a man's genitals or examine the prostate through the rectum. In most cases, most physicians do not even ask questions about the patient's sex life, which could provide clues to physical disorders. This reality for men is in stark contrast to the rigorous yearly exams that most women undergo with their gynecologists. The fact that doctors do not examine men on a regular basis is a major contributing factor to the widespread ignorance I have witnessed in men with regard to awareness of their bodies in general and their genitals specifically.

For urologists, by far the most common male problem we see is enlargement of the prostate. For that reason, all men over forty should insist on a digital prostate exam when they have their physicals (which is not a computerized process, but rather a rectal exam done by the gloved finger or "digit" of the examining physician). I know this procedure can be uncomfortable and embarrassing. It is a small price to pay for detecting the early warning signs of trouble. It is well-established that the early diagnosis of prostate cancer has an extremely high success rate of restoring prostate health. If a prostate cancer is still confined within the prostate and has not extended beyond the "capsule," prompt, early treatment offers a high percentage of disease-free survival. Early diagnosis is the key. If you experience any of the following symptoms, you should seek an immediate urologic consultation:

- A weak or interrupted urinary stream
- Difficulty starting the urinary stream
- The need to urinate frequently, especially throughout the night

- Blood in the urine
- Dribbling after you think you have completely emptied your bladder
- Painful or burning urination (dysuria)
- Persistent pain in the lower back, pelvis, or lower abdomen

Bear in mind that we now have many sophisticated, noninvasive tests for diagnosing prostate disease. The transrectal ultrasonic probe, which is only about as uncomfortable as a rectal thermometer, has revolutionized diagnosis. Using sound waves, like the sonar in a submarine, the probe enables us to determine the volume of the prostate gland and view its internal structure. Pictures can be filed in the patient's record for comparison during subsequent exams. The test alerts us to abnormalities that could be signs of prostate disease, including cancer.

Another, even more important revolution in the diagnosis of prostate cancer is the prostate specific antigen blood test, or PSA, the male equivalent of the Pap smear and mammogram in women. This is a routine, painless way to potentially detect cancer in time to treat it effectively. Men produce a specific antigen in response to prostate cancer. The measurement of the PSA volume in circulating blood tells us if the antigen is present at abnormal levels. If it is, we use ultrasound technology to locate the tumor focus and then precisely biopsy the specific area—all in about one minute—without making any incision in the skin. I strongly recommend a PSA test as part of a routine annual screening for men over forty-five, although it is not a bad idea to start at forty. I cannot emphasize this point enough: mounting evidence indicates that the *early diagnosis and treatment of prostate cancer saves patients lives!*

You may be wondering why I have not described what the mechanisms and causes of prostate cancer may be. Although a number of theories have attempted to explain how and why this deadly disease comes about, not enough scientific and medical evidence is available at this time to identify a definitive cause. Some studies have indicated that heredity is a major factor in the development of prostate disease. For example, those men who have a blood relative (e.g., a father or a brother) who has had prostate cancer before turning sixty are 50 percent more likely to develop the disease than the average man.[2] If two blood relatives have had the disease (e.g., a father *and* a brother), it is about two and a half times more likely that he will get the disease.[3] Other studies have shown that the rate of incidence is also related to race. Prostate cancer has been found to be highest among African Americans and lowest among Asians. Surprisingly, studies show a low rate of incidence among Africans. Since African Americans share some genetic lineage with Africans, this difference suggests that dietary and lifestyle habits can play a role in the development of prostate cancer. Although much of this research is still in a preliminary phase, the anecdotal evidence gives some indication that prostate cancer is related to both genes and lifestyle.

With regard to the prevention of prostate problems, I have one suggestion in addition to regular examinations: *have a lot of sex.* Like all organs, the prostate benefits from exercise, and the best exercise it can get is ejaculation. When you ejaculate, your perineal muscles contract violently (the band of muscles that make up the perineum, the space between the rectum and the base of the testicle). This provides a massage of sorts for the prostate gland, which keeps its ducts open and prevents its internal fluids from becoming stagnant.

New technology now enables us to detect various tumors in the urinary bladder or testicles at an early stage. The treatment of testicular cancer has vastly improved over the past few years. In 1963, 63 percent of patients suffering from testicular cancer survived; now, more than 95 percent are curable[4] (see the Lance Armstrong story in chapter 5).

Unlike prostate cancer, testicular cancer occurs mainly in men under forty. Regardless of your age, however, I strongly suggest that you self-examine your testicles monthly and feel for suspicious lumps (and also educate your male children as well). Just as doctors recommend that women (from teenage years on) examine their breasts for lumps to screen for breast cancer, men need to examine their testicles. The more often you examine yourself, the more familiar you will become with the structure of your testicles and the more equipped you will be to detect any abnormalities. The best time for self-examination is after a warm bath or shower when the scrotum is relaxed. Your testicles should feel like hard-boiled eggs without the shells: smooth and void of lumps. Any lump, even a painless one, should be reported to your doctor immediately. You may palpate an abnormality during self-examination or your sexual partner may notice it while making love. In either case, further evaluation by your urologist is a must. (Incidentally, if you notice that one of your testes is lower than the other, do not panic. One testis is *always* lower. It is nature's way of making sure those two sources of life do not crash into one another—a design for which all men should be grateful!)

Finally, if you ever experience a *sudden* onset of penis weakness, you should first rule out all possible *physical* causes by seeing a doctor immediately. If you do not have a doctor who examines your genitals, or if your doctor is someone with whom you are not comfortable discussing your sexual well-being, then you should try to find one who understands that your sexual organs are not merely machines that perform biological services. A good doctor comprehends that the penis is not just a functional body part but also a psychological and spiritual agent designed to bring you pleasure. Your doctor should be someone with whom you feel comfortable sharing the intimate details of your life. If this is not the case, then the time may be right for a visit to your local urologist.

Part 2

Becoming a Superpotent Man

Chapter 13

What's Your Penis Personality?

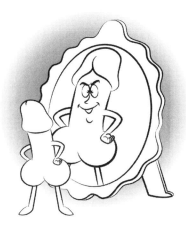

Most people's opinion of the penis can pretty much be summed up in the age-old saying "It has a mind of its own." This is one of those classic clichés I constantly hear from my patients and friends in reference to their penises. This statement reflects the issues surrounding what I call the *penis mystique*.

One of the reasons we are so fascinated by that "junior partner," as a lawyer patient of mine calls his, is that it *does* seem to think for itself. What other organ grows to several times its normal size and then shrinks again, sometimes despite our intentions and without warning? What other organ is so unpredictable?

That's why we speak about it, and maybe even speak *to* it, as if it were a person. Men say, "My penis did this or my penis did that," as if it makes its own decisions. However much your penis appears to act on its own, your penis is not separate from your self.

The penis does not have a mind of its own. In fact, it reads your mind. It not only reads your mind, it reads your *heart* and *soul* as well. The behavior of your penis is a very accurate reflection of your state of being. At any given moment, it reflects your thoughts and feelings more accurately than any other part of your body.

When you are up, so is your penis.

When you are down, your penis will be down as well.

When you feel strong, vigorous, creative, and confident, your penis is strong, vigorous, creative, and confident, too.

When you feel tired, apathetic, depressed, or impatient, your penis is also tired, apathetic, depressed, and impatient. The connection between the mind and the penis is one of the most powerful forces in the complex structure of male sexuality.

The reason the penis seems to have a mind of its own and sometimes acts contrary to your wishes is because even though you may not always be in touch with what you are really thinking and feeling, your penis *is* in touch. Through a vast network of nerves and blood vessels, the penis has a direct connection to your brain.

You cannot fool it.

If you are angry, nervous, or worried and try to hide your feelings by putting on a happy, sexy exterior, your penis will not only know the truth, but it will also reveal the truth by its behavior.

If your partner offends you or hurts you, you can bet that, no matter how hard you try to conceal your feelings, your penis will act hurt and offended. On the contrary, if your partner adores you, flatters you, and wants you, your penis will respond positively, even if you do not think you are in the mood.

The behavior of your penis is a more accurate barometer of what you are feeling at any particular moment than your own conscious assessment.

Like the eyes, the penis is an organ of expression. It embodies a man's personality. That is why, over the many years I have examined penises and talked to the men to whom they are attached, I have observed a definite correlation between how men behave sexually and how they behave in general. Men who have a negative penis image tend to have a poor self-image overall, while men with a positive penis image tend to see themselves in a positive light. For the most part, we behave in the bedroom much the same way we behave in the living room, boardroom, factory, gym, or driving on the freeway.

In the rest of this chapter, I will describe some of the Penis Personalities I have met in more than thirty years practicing urology. These Penis Personalities are not mutually exclusive. Any man might exhibit several of them, or he may shift from one to another depending on circumstances.

It is also important to note that these personality traits are not exclusive to the penis. This chapter could just as easily be called "Vagina Personalities." The traits apply to women just the same as they do to men.

The link between self-image and sexual identity is a critical point from which much of sexual weakness or sexual power stems. In order to better understand this correlation, the following section examines the psychological traits of certain personality types and how those traits relate to sexuality. You will want to see which ones fit you and which ones do not. You will decide which traits you want to adopt and which traits you may need to reject. You may even have some fun categorizing your friends' Penis Personalities. Try to approach this section with an open mind and a willingness to examine yourself with the honest intent of improving who you are both as a person and as a sexual being.

Let's begin with positive Penis Personalities. These are traits worthy of admiration. Every man should aspire to these traits. He should do all he can to emulate them.

Positive Penis Personalities

The Purposeful Penis Personality

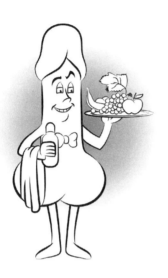

The Purposeful Penis Personality approaches sex with his partner's satisfaction as his highest priority. He studies his partner's behavior, learns the nuanced intricacies of her desires, and applies his experience and skills to the fulfillment of those desires. The Purposeful Penis is a great student of love. He is thorough in his self-education and applies all that he has learned to the specific needs of his lover. His knowledge is always balanced by an educated sensitivity.

The Perceptive Penis Personality

The Perceptive Penis Personality is an understanding man with an understanding penis. He empathizes with his partner. He responds generously to his partner's needs and intuitively picks up on unexpressed moods and desires. It is as if his penis were a submarine periscope poking its head above the surface into the light. In that light, the Perceptive Penis assesses the psychological atmosphere and always strives to make the best possible decisions.

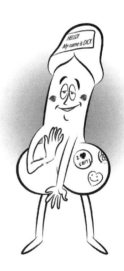

The Persistent Penis Personality

The Persistent Penis Personality does not accept defeat. When he desires someone, he will pursue that person with determination. He will never allow self-doubt or fear to weaken his drive. He pursues intelligently, diplomatically, and persuasively. He is not a pest, a harasser, or a date rapist. In bed, he aims for a level of performance and fulfillment that he and his partner both desire. His persistence is defined by grace and style. His attitude is character-

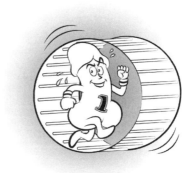

ized by confidence *and* understanding. He knows how to get what he wants.

The Principled Penis Personality

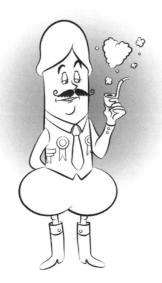

The Principled Penis Personality holds honor and integrity as the highest standards for love. His unyielding personal standards of right and wrong guide his sexual behavior in every encounter. He is a classic gentleman. His every romantic action is dictated by respect, sensibility, and consideration for the dignity of his partner. This man is the embodiment of all that is good about love.

The Percolating Penis Personality

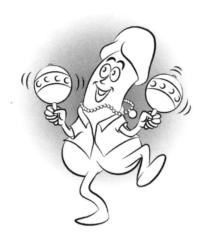

The Percolating Penis Personality is always cooking. He is always ready for action. He is positive. His positive outlook bubbles over. Regardless of his age, he is dynamic, youthful, and energetic. He enjoys attention and seeks it out but does so in a likable manner. He is endearing without arrogance or bravado. People like a man with this personality. He is fun and exciting, and his percolating penis reheats quickly.

The Prepared Penis Personality

The man with a Prepared Penis Personality is more than just a "condom bearer" or a bedroom boy scout. He is a lover who is equipped with a warm fire. He has a glass of water or wine when thirst prevails. He has a warm smile and a hug when sensitivity is needed. He is a lover who is prepared for anything that may come his way. If the Prepared Penis is confronted with a hurdle for which he is *not* prepared, he proves himself as a man of wit and creative charm. He goes the extra mile to make every moment perfect.

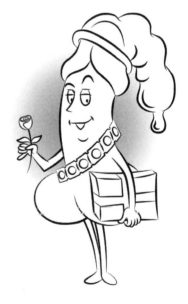

The Pensive Penis Personality

A cartoonist would portray the Pensive Penis Personality in a tweed condom and horn-rimmed glasses. The Pensive Penis likes to think things through. He is intelligent, well informed, and clear thinking about sex and his partner. He strives to be knowledgeable. He studies as much as he can about sex and is always probing for fresh ways to bring pleasure to his lover. There is a caveat for the Pensive Penis. If he gets *too* calculating, he can miss out on a lot of fun because he's *thinking* when he ought to be *feeling*.

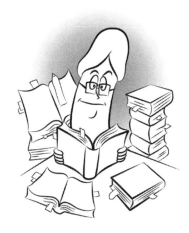

The Philanthropic Penis Personality

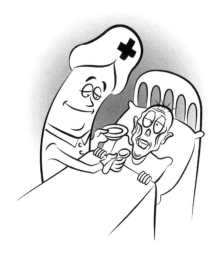

The Philanthropic Penis Personality is a good-hearted soul who finds nothing more satisfying than giving pleasure to his partner. When not involved in a long-term relationship, he is drawn to people in need of comfort or solace. He is drawn to the romantic types who have been hurt by callousness and who yearn for someone who is generous and caring. He gives his partners an emotionally rich sexual experience. But he has to beware of being so concerned about his partner's fulfillment that he neglects his own desires and needs.

The Protective Penis Personality

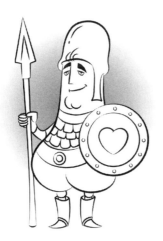

The Protective Penis Personality is the "gentle lover." For him, every act is centered on his partner's emotional and physical security. In his arms, any lover would feel safe from the evils of the world. He has the unique ability to create the environment in which vulnerable partners can fully express themselves without fear. He is not aggressive or violently possessive. He merely emits an aura of strength and security. He always defends the well-being of his partner both physically and emotionally.

The Passionate Penis Personality

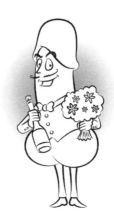

Rhett Butler and Prince Charming or George Clooney and Brad Pitt are the Passionate Penis Personality's role models. This gentleman is a lover's lover with boundless enthusiasm for life. Emotional, ardent, and lusty, he likes grand gestures and noble statements. He sends bouquets. He showers his lover with compliments. He waxes poetic. He dances cheek to cheek, and he always means it. He remembers birthdays and anniversaries, and if he forgets, he will make up for his error magnificently. He is likely to have a clever nickname for his penis, something like "Lancelot." He regards his penis as a staunch friend and trusted ally in the service of l'amour. Lovers find him irresistible because he is as sensitive as he is strong.

The Psychedelic Penis Personality

The Psychedelic Penis Personality is wild and experimental. I refer to him as the "polytechnic" Penis Personality. With this lover, the sexual experience becomes a wonderful mix of heightened effects. Every moment is a vibrant swirl of colors, sounds, and emotional excitement. He takes sex *beyond* reality by adding new dimensions to old habits while maintaining the respect and sensitivity of a sane lover. He achieves all of this with the genius of his own skill and imagination. He does not rely on drugs or illicit substances.

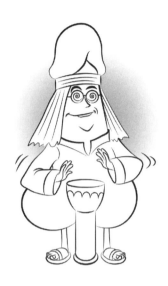

The Peaceful Penis Personality

The Peaceful Penis Personality is a calm man whose penis is relaxed—in the psychological sense. The Peaceful Penis has a sexuality that is raring to go but presents itself with a cool, collected dignity. He is not complacent. He simply does not demand much and is able to extract great pleasure from whatever life places before him. He is a gentle, tender lover, but behind that tenderness is great passion.

The Pioneer Penis Personality

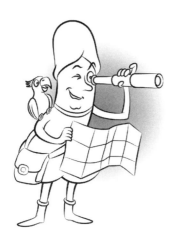

For the Pioneer Penis Personality, versatility is his name and imagination is his game. The Pioneer Penis is a trailblazer. He will try anything new in the spirit of adventure and fun. He adapts to unexpected conditions easily and eagerly. Perhaps it is a tryst, a partner who is more voracious (or more reluctant) than he anticipated, or an unlikely location. He is at home in a lavatory in an airplane (the "mile high" club) or in a broom closet. As one of my patients told me, "If oranges are in demand on Tuesday, you'd better have oranges for sale. If on Wednesday everyone wants bananas, you'd better get a truckload of bananas." This is the kind of lover who satisfies a partner with new, exciting, and innovative approaches to love.

The Playful Penis Personality

Meet the party guy: upbeat, festive, and maybe a little bit mischievous. The Playful Penis Personality is full of surprises. He might swoop down on his lover when least expected. He may show up at her office and whisk her off to a hotel for the afternoon. If penises were automobiles, his would be a sports car. This personality is always ready to laugh. He never takes himself or his penis too seriously. He might tell a joke in the middle of making love and not miss a beat. For this guy, his own funny bone is an erogenous zone. To him, a partner with a sense of humor has the sex appeal of a centerfold.

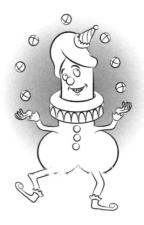

The Precocious Penis Personality

The Precocious Penis Personality is the young man who is sexually aware at an early age. He knows what to do and how to do it long before his peers. If he is mature enough to approach sex responsibly, he might be so active that it drives his buddies wild with envy. He does not have a shy bone in his body, nor does he have a shy *boner*. Older women might feel guilty about the feelings this character arouses in them. He may not be

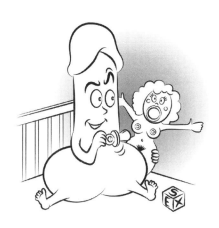

good-looking. He has that certain something that comes from his penis confidence. Keep in mind that precocity is not limited to the very young. When a mature man is up-front and very personal, he can be just as precocious as a youth. The Precocious Penis makes his intentions known. This is a trait that can be obnoxious in the wrong hands but is charming in his. Women might be shocked for a moment, but they quickly recover and find him refreshingly direct.

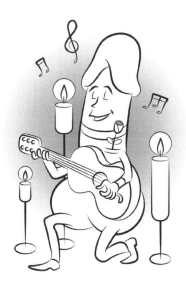

The Poetic Penis Personality

The Poetic Penis Personality has a thoughtful and imaginative sensibility. He speaks a language of love filled with deep thought, feeling, and life experience. This lover is sensitive to the needs of his partner. He makes every experience a romantic tour de force. He knows how to cajole his partner using the right words or actions. He always means what he says and does. He makes love like a dancer, with poetry and precision in his every movement.

The Prodigious Penis Personality

The Prodigious Penis Personality may not be prodigiously large, but he thinks and acts as if he is. This man not only has a bustling libido, he also has an abundant heart and a generous soul. He sees himself as possessing great bounty and he gives of himself freely. He knows that he will be replenished in return. He is ready for sex at any time and in any place. He has what I call *penis largesse*. He can extract maximum pleasure from any situation. Women are drawn to him, sometimes for reasons they cannot explain.

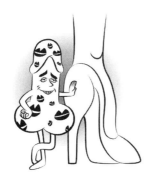

The Powerful Penis Personality

Penis power does not come from arriving at the party in a fancy car, having the biggest bank account, or parading around town in an expensive power suit. The Powerful Penis exudes a sexual control from within. This may be displayed by the quiet and commanding confidence of a simple glance or an engaging smile that says, "Have no fear, power is here!" His internal control is accompanied by a body language that exudes power and safety. In the bedroom, this personality takes command

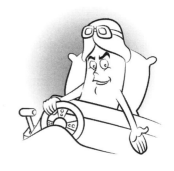

with the authority of a master conductor. He achieves the fullest expression of every instrument in an orchestra. He commands with the confidence of experience and knowledge, illuminating the deep language of the sexual experience. This lover has a strong effect, both physically and emotionally.

These Positive Penis Personalities represent those positive traits that all men and women should strive to attain. They have qualities that will help enable any lover to achieve his personal goals, both in the bedroom and in life. All of these characteristics are embodied in the ultimate Penis Personality: the *superpotent man*.

Negative Penis Personalities

Now let us take a look at the other side of the fence at what, in my clinical judgment, are negative Penis Personalities. *Negative Penis Personalities are the sources of penis weakness. These personalities are to be avoided at all costs.* If you find that these descriptions match your personality and character, then overcoming these traits should be the highest priority in your quest toward the full expression of your penis power.

The Peewee Penis Personality

The Peewee Penis Personality *thinks* small. He perceives his penis as undersized or inadequate. He sees himself as a small man. He may try to overcompensate by being a shark in business or by driving fancy cars, but these superficial defense mechanisms mean nothing. He views himself and his penis through the wrong end of a telescope. This man develops a weak and fearful personality. Ironically, chances are unlikely that his penis is smaller than normal.

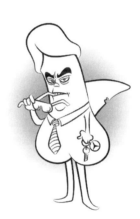

The Pessimistic Penis Personality

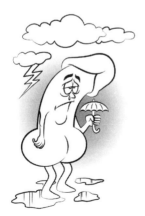

The Pessimistic Penis Personality is a downer. He is a glass that is always half empty. He approaches every activity in his life with the preconceived notion that it won't work out. This includes his sexual activity. He believes that if he does manage to get a woman into bed, his penis won't be big enough or hard enough or that he won't last long enough. His gloomy predictions usually turn out to be right. He has doomed himself psychologically.

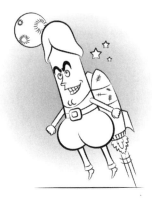

The Promiscuous Penis Personality

The Promiscuous Penis Personality is always on the lookout for new conquests. He is very insecure. He needs to carve notches on his belt, even if he's married. In this age of AIDS, this indiscriminate character is a dangerous man. Nothing is wrong with being sexually adventurous. However, I advise patients who are ready to plug themselves into any socket at any time like an appliance that discretion in new sexual relationships will bring less trouble and more pleasure in the long run.

The Procrastinating Penis Personality

Why have sex here and now when you can put it off until tomorrow? That is what the Procrastinating Penis thinks. It is never the right time, place, or partner. If he wants someone, he will put off contacting her for so long that she will probably forget who he is. The procrastinator is not lazy; he is simply scared. He is so terrified of penis failure that he cannot bring himself to face the challenge.

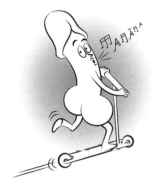

The Phobic Penis Personality

Imagine a penis huddling fearfully inside a pair of pants and peeking through the zipper to make sure it is safe to come out. If you can picture this, you can envision the Phobic Penis Personality. This personality has irrational phobias. He may have an aversion to certain smells, to pubic hair, to large breasts, to unlocked bedrooms, or even to the dark. He might be petrified of disease—not just of the HIV-retrovirus but also of any conceivable germ in any environment. He might be terrified of vaginas, fearing that one will ensnare him like a Venus flytrap. Any kind of irrational fear will keep this man from enjoying sex as surely as an arachnophobe avoids spiders.

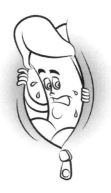

The Picky Penis Personality

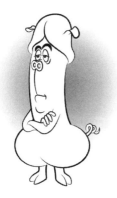

The Picky Penis Personality is so obstinate and narrow-minded that he takes all the enjoyment out of using his penis. Everything has to be "just so" before he can function properly. His partner has to be *this* size and *that* shape. His partner has to do things his way. He is responsive only to a narrow range of turnons. He rarely compromises. When I see him as a patient, I see a pigheaded man. "Don't confuse me with the facts—my mind is already made up" is his attitude, even about his own health.

The Pile-Driver Penis Personality

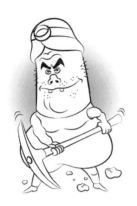

The Pile-Driver Penis Personality is a bulldozer type who approaches vaginas like a violent jackhammer. "Wham, bam, thank you, ma'am" typifies his character. Crude and clumsy, he has no time for romance or foreplay. He pounds, plunges, and jabs. Sometimes he injures his partners. He is not vicious or sadistic. He might be a pussycat, but when he is aroused, look out! If he is lucky, he will hook up with someone who enjoys his approach. There is, indeed, someone for nearly everyone! Any person who finds themselves with a Pile Driver is well advised to settle him down before he gets into bed. That is, of course, unless you enjoy feeling like a trampoline.

The Petulant Penis Personality

Rude and insolent, the contentious Petulant Penis Personality wants to stick his penis where it is not wanted or where it is not ready to be received. He has to have everything his way. If his partner hesitates to meet his demands, he acts as if he's being "put on." If things do not work out for him, the other person is always at fault. He hurts others and ultimately hurts himself.

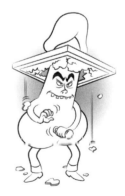

The Pornographic Penis Personality

As a way of occasionally enhancing a relationship, pornography can be useful and fun. The Pornographic Penis *needs* erotic material to get aroused. To him, a warm body is not as stimulating as a moving picture or an erotic passage from a book. My attitude is whatever turns you on as long as it is safe and legal is acceptable, medically and ethically. However, I always advise my patients to make the most of reality instead of relying too much on fantasy.

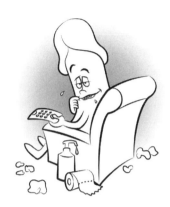

The Plaintiff Penis Personality

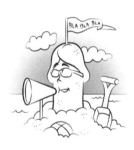

The Plaintiff Penis Personality adds up what he gets and what he gives. He evaluates the totals according to his version of justice. I am in favor of fair play when it comes to sex. However, the guy with the Plaintiff Personality has his own code and his own method of calculating. When he comes up short, he litigates: "I did this and that for you. Now you have to do X, Y, and Z for me." To my amazement, actual litigation sometimes arises. One of my patients took his wife to court for denying him his right to more and better sex. She countersued, claiming he had let himself go physically and was a chronic premature ejaculator. If this sounds like you, take it easy or you may find yourself behind the bars of sexual loneliness.

The Pompous Penis Personality

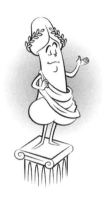

Every man should have penis pride but the Pompous Penis Personality is narcissistic. He is the locker-room braggart who spins crude tales about his conquests and his prodigious feats. Even if his exploits are true, his manner is so offensive that listeners conclude he is a phony. Just as millionaires with class do not boast about their wealth, men of true penis power do not brag about their sexual accomplishments.

This arrogant, self-important individual misrepresents himself to his partners. He promises a night of bliss but often falls short of his boastful arrogance. The penis is a great equalizer. It is the most honest part of a man's anatomy. It cannot lie. It reveals its own character as well as the personality flaws of its owner. Be cautious with your arrogance. You may be the only one left to listen to your own bravado.

The Pipe-Dream Penis Personality

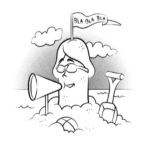

Like a perpetual adolescent, the Pipe-Dream Penis Personality lives in a world where he is a combination of Tommy Lee and Ron Jeremy—a world in which flawless women lust for him and he satisfies their every desire. The only satisfactory sex he has is above the neck. His mind is XXX-rated, but his penis is strictly Family Channel.

When I encounter such men, I try to convince them to be proud of what God has given them. If they use what they have intelligently, and if they accept the real sexual opportunities before them with gratitude, they do not have to live in a fantasy world.

The Pious Penis Personality

The Pious Penis Personality could be a minister, priest, rabbi, or mullah. He could even be a devout layman trying to conform to scripture. Men who abstain from sex because of religious beliefs tend to be torn by conflict. As a scientist, it is hard for me to comprehend how a man can restrain a normal sex drive without suffering debilitating consequences. Physiologically, these men have the same needs as everyone else. Nevertheless, many pious men are able to keep their penises under wraps. They manage to maintain vows while exhibiting a sense of joy and a tolerance for those with more liberal attitudes. These men deserve and receive my respect. But the man who struggles to repress his sexuality and who resents having to bear that burden is to be pitied. The pious hypocrite who cavorts with hookers or molests young children while threatening "sinners" with fire and damnation deserves neither respect nor pity.

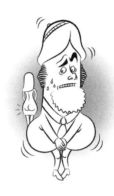

The Pedestrian Penis Personality

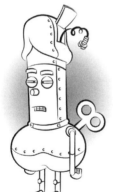

The missionary position is the most adventurous escapade for the Pedestrian Penis Personality. He is unimaginative, mechanical, and without spontaneity. He is the sexual equivalent of an automatic camera that does everything it is programmed to do. He is a man of highly regimented routines. If his partner suggests catching a later train and grabbing a quickie in the kitchen, he thinks she has been reading too many romance novels. I try, usually in vain, to get these guys to loosen up before they find themselves sexually dried up and sometimes divorced or single.

The Political Penis Personality

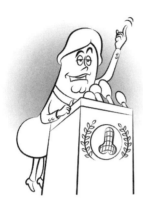

A chameleon with an unerring knack for telling you what you want to hear by speaking with equal conviction out of both sides of his mouth, the Political Penis alters his character to suit each potential constituent. He seldom lives up to his campaign promises. If this type is in a position of power, he will not hesitate to use his status to service his penis. He will never fail to use his penis to improve his position. If he could sleep his way to the top, he would be delighted. If he could get a gullible, ambitious woman into the sack by promising her a seat on the fast track or by threatening to demote her to the caboose, he would not hesitate for a second. To him, sexual harassment is just part of the law of the jungle.

The Pooped Penis Personality

Ho hum! The Pooped Penis Personality needs a long vacation. He is tired, burned out, and limp, and so is his penis. More people complain to me of this syndrome than any other. These men are middle-aged, overworked, stressed-out professionals: lawyers, executives, even some of my medical colleagues. They work too many hours, shoulder too many burdens, and leave no time or energy for the oldest and simplest form of rejuvenation—sex. If there was a way to make love while mingling with movers and shakers, schmoozing a client, or closing a deal, they would do it more often. By the time they get

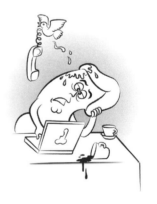

home to their partners, they can barely raise their fingers, let alone their penises. I tell these men, "If you're too busy for sex, you are *simply* too busy!"

The Preoccupied Penis Personality

When the Pooped Penis Personality is not pooped, he is preoccupied. This guy makes love on automatic pilot. His mind is always someplace other than where it belongs. His mind should be focused on his penis, his lips, his hands, and where on his lover's body these parts happen to be. Instead, his mind is at the office or at the ball game, and he is missing out on the best nontelevised sport in the world.

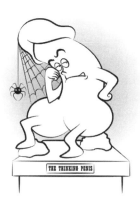

THE THINKING PENIS

The Paranoid Penis Personality

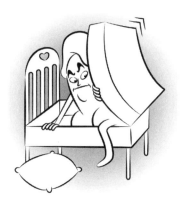

The Paranoid Penis Personality is suspicious that if someone is willing to go to bed with him she must have ulterior motives. "What does she *really* want?" he wonders. If he can get over that hurdle, he will worry about whatever else it is about his partner that strikes him as threatening. His lover can show him personalized data from the Centers for Disease Control, and he will still worry about the germs he might pick up. He thinks God made sexually transmitted diseases just to get him. Unfortunately, anyone who is as fearful as this guy will never live up to his own sexual capacity.

The Pampered Penis Personality

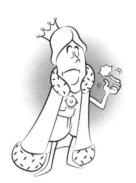

The Pampered Penis Personality is a prima donna who feels entitled to special treatment. You expect his penis to stand up and sing something like the song from *Funny Girl*—"Do things for me, buy things for me, cater to my every whim." I believe the penis *should* be fussed over. It *should* be the center of attention. But demanding to be pampered without offering reciprocation or gratitude is not a sign of positive penis power—it is a sign of insecure neediness.

The Pissed-Off Penis Personality

The Pissed-Off Penis is angry at the world. He is angry at love. He cannot stand rejection. He cannot stand honest emotions. When things go wrong, it is everyone's fault *but his*. Sexually, his hostility can express itself in a number of ways. He might satisfy himself without reciprocating for his partner. He might force his partner to do things she does not want to do. He might promise whatever it takes to get someone into bed, then flaunt his lies and leave. He might intentionally hurt his partner and act as though it were an accident.

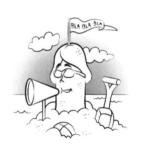

In a healthy relationship, sex can sometimes be a perfect and natural way to release tension and work off stress. But sex should never be an outlet for anger and frustration. I advise my patients to avoid becoming the type of man for whom sex is an expression of hostility. I advise everyone to steer clear of this potentially hurtful character.

The Profligate Penis Personality

There is no way you can wear out your penis by using it for its intended purpose. You can damage other parts of your body and other parts of your life by overindulging your penis. The Profligate Penis Personality is given to dissipation. He is extravagant and wildly self-indulgent. These are relative terms. What is profligate for an older or ailing man might be harmless excitement for a young, healthy guy. But when you follow your penis to the point of not eating or sleeping properly, or your sexual exploits jeopardize your job or family, then you have gone too far.

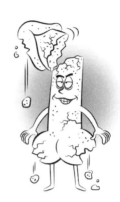

The Possessive Penis Personality

"If you sleep with me, I own you." That's the attitude of the Possessive Penis Personality. He does not want a lover; he wants an emotional and physical slave. Making some demands and insisting on fidelity are not signs of weakness, but this type wants to dominate and control his partner's life and every aspect of her sexuality to an unhealthy degree.

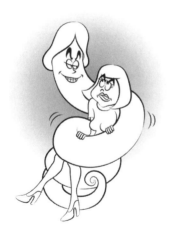

The Perverted Penis Personality

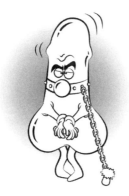

It is not my job to label any sexual act as a perversion. One person's perversion is another one's pleasure. As long as no one is being hurt or abused, I have no ethical or medical objection to any act between consenting adults. I have observed the Perverted Penis Personality as a character that is only drawn to acts that are on the edge. He is aroused by things that make most people cringe. His partner usually has to be seduced or coerced into joining him. He reminds me of the wife in Woody Allen's *Everything You Always Wanted to Know about Sex (But Were Afraid to Ask)*, who could only have sex in public places where there was a risk of being seen. The danger for this personality is never being satisfied with partners who may be a positive match for a healthy emotional relationship. Most people with these radical tastes prevent many potentially positive relationships from developing. These relationships are spoiled because partners are deterred by these strange and sometimes offensive sexual practices. It is important to express yourself and to do what pleases you most. I must advise that doing so at the cost of your happiness is foolish.

The Professional Penis Personality

The Professional Penis Personality is the prostitute and the gigolo, unhealthy but interesting. The man who has the Professional Penis Personality is confident in his sexuality. This confidence extends to a dangerous level. He knows how to exert his power. This type of lifestyle usually leads to a never-ending string of bad relationships, both professionally and personal. The Professional Penis creates an unhealthy connection to sex in particular and to love in general. With all of the health hazards of reckless sexual intercourse, these individuals put themselves and their partners at great risk. Selling one's sex can cause permanent damage to both the psychological and emotional health of the person who chooses this unfortunate path.

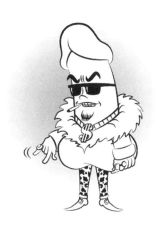

I also place the pimp and procurer in this category. I have treated a number of pimps over the years. Although their behavior is reprehensible, I have found them fascinating individuals. They have an uncanny ability to mesmerize women. Despite suffering extreme mistreatment and exploitation, their women seem to enjoy bringing home money and having sex with them after a long night of servicing clients. Anyone who finds that he is swept up in the slick style of these hustlers should find every possible way out before it is too late. Dealing with these men, I often find myself wishing that their positive penis attitude could be transmitted to men who would make better use of it.

The Pharmaceutical Penis Personality

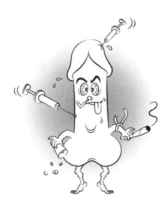

Some men need to medicate themselves before they can have satisfactory sex. That typically entails a few drinks, a tranquilizer, or a few tokes of marijuana to loosen their inhibitions. Others do not think they *need* drugs, but they prefer using them. They turn to chemicals for heightened sensation. It does not matter whether the drug of choice is cocaine, amphetamines, crystal meth, or amyl-nitrate. The Pharmaceutical Penis Personality is likely to become dependent on substances with harmful side effects. In the long term, men with this personality have their penis power debilitated, along with their general health. I try to convince them that the benefits of drugs and excessive alcohol are illusory and that they can function perfectly well without that assistance.

The same also goes for the blatant abuse of erectile dysfunction medication such as Viagra, Levitra, or Cialis. Recently, it has come to my attention that many men who are *not* prescribed these very potent drugs have begun experimenting with the use of these medications in intimate sexual encounters and even at sex parties and orgies. I discuss the potentially dangerous effects of these vasoactive, performance-enhancing drugs in chapter 6, "Blue Pills and Other Medical Cures for Erectile Dysfunction." It should serve as a reminder to any man who strives to become superpotent that abusing prescription medication can be *just as dangerous and potentially harmful* to penis power as abusing illicit substances.

As a general rule, any man with true penis power should avoid illicit drugs. When prescribed by a knowledgeable physician, the use of Viagra, Cialis, and Levitra can be safe and effective.

Reducing the number and intensity of these negative traits and emulating the Positive Penis Personalities is the goal to which I would like to see all men aspire. If you follow the advice in the rest of this book, that is precisely what you will achieve.

The characteristics discussed in this chapter are universal. They apply to both men and women. They are a wonderful point of departure for discussions between partners. They can be a very useful communication tool to break the ice with what is usually an uncomfortable subject. I urge all of my readers to take the necessary time to reflect on which of these personality traits, both positive and negative, they and their partners might have.

If you are being held back by some of the negative characteristics, then overcoming their stifling effect should be of the utmost priority. If you or your partner has some of these negative qualities and they are having a harmful effect on your relationship, talk about it openly. Be honest with yourself. Recognize the areas in your personality that may need some adjustment. Help your partner to acknowledge whatever issues she may have with herself, so that ultimately your relationship can reach its greatest potential. The future of your personal and sexual happiness rests on these fundamental psychological issues. To become a man of true penis power, you must have the courage and strength to change what is not working and create a path of change that leads to *superpotency*.

Chapter 14

What Is a Superpotent Man?

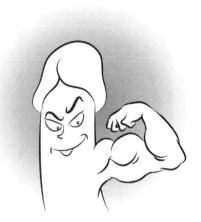

I have been privy to the intimate details of hundreds of thousands of patients' lives. I have analyzed their physical health, their mental health, their business life, and their social life. In addition, other men and women—colleagues, friends, and family members—have taken advantage of my professional status and my medical curiosity to discuss their sex lives. I have come to develop the portrait of a special Penis Personality that is worthy of its own chapter: the Superpotent Man.

Superpotency is a birthright. It should be seen as a natural state of affairs, not as an exception. Every man can learn to harness its power. Every man can reap its great rewards. As I describe the attributes that define this character, you might find yourself thinking, "I cannot be like that. I'll never be that kind of guy." I can only say: "Nonsense!"

This is just the kind of negative thinking that prevents you from expressing all of your potential. By the time you finish this book, you should be well on your way. Superpotency is a process that begins with thinking positively about yourself, your penis, and your sexuality.

Discovering Penis Power

Some men command attention. You have seen them before. They fill the room and turn heads. They are magnetic. Strong and confident men view them with admiration and respect. Weaker men are awestruck or intimidated.

People recognize an inherent power in these types of men—a power that emanates from something greater than money, prestige, or looks. Many tend to be attracted to these individuals, both physically and mentally. If these people are in the market for sex or romance, they are top candidates. These men have that certain "something." You might call it presence. You might call it sex appeal. You might just call it "It." I call it *penis power*.

Penis power is not about looks or status. It is especially not about penis size. Superpotent men are not necessarily handsome. They do not have to be hunks, and they would not necessarily pass an audition for a beefcake calendar.

There are handsome men with penis power and handsome men without it. The same is true for the guys who people may think are unattractive. The guy who has both looks and superpotency has a lot going for him. But between a handsome man without it and a homely man with it, the latter of the two will attract more partners and will lead a more satisfying life.

Take a look at some of the famous movie stars who are considered sexy even though they are not blessed with classic good looks. Look at the French actor Gerard Depardieu and the American actor Owen Wilson. They are both average-looking men with doughy faces and oversized noses. Yet there is no denying their sex appeal. I do not know either of them, but I would be willing to wager they possess abundant penis power. That is not just because of their celebrity lifestyle.

How about Jack Nicholson? He is balding, potbellied, and has wild eyebrows and a face no Greek sculptor would use as a model. But he has something that women *and* men find irresistible. There is also the famous example of the film producer Carlo Ponti. Forty years ago, he was a small, bald, ordinary-looking man. He was the last man you would expect to see with a gorgeous, talented, voluptuous, sexy woman. To everyone's surprise, Ponti married the most desired woman in the world at that time—Sophia Loren. And she *stayed* married to him.

On the flip side, there are also many examples of gorgeous hunks who satisfy every aesthetic criterion but who do not arouse attention. These men are not necessarily sexy.

I remember one day when a patient walked into my office. He was an incredible physical specimen. He was a professional athlete with a body of solid muscle and a face you would expect to see on the cover of *GQ*. I assumed he was the kind of guy who had girls falling at his feet. So I teased the women in my office by asking which ones would like to meet him. There were no takers. I was shocked and surprised when one of the women explained, "It's all on the outside. He just doesn't have *it*."

These stories demonstrate that *superpotency is not about looks*. If you develop the self-confidence and strength that are the foundation of penis power, you will find that you look much better in your mind's eye. Any man who desires this power will take responsibility for his physical appearance by maintaining a healthy diet and a healthy regimen of exercise. Ultimately, by making the necessary changes in lifestyle and perspective, those physical attributes that may have been a source of self-doubt in the past will suddenly have more appeal.

Superpotency is not about wealth or social position. Superpotent men tend to be relatively successful in their chosen fields because their personal qualities foster achievement. However, being a man of wealth and status does not qualify you as superpotent. I cannot deny the fact that many people are attracted to rich and power-ful men just because they are rich and powerful. But the appeal of wealth and status is a superficial appeal and, nine times out of ten, this superficiality does not translate into genuine qualities worthy of admiration.

Once the fancy car is parked in its Beverly Hills garage, the $3,000 suit is hung in the closet, and the silk underwear is removed, the rich man might be much less potent than the struggling artist in his garret or the assembly-line worker in his tract home.

Penis power comes from within. The only form of abundance that really counts is an *attitude* of abundance—an attitude of self-confidence and control toward oneself and one's sexuality.

My patients and acquaintances are some of the richest and most influential people in the world. Many of these men have true penis power. A far greater number have power in their offices, but they are plagued by penis weakness. They have personal insecurities in their minds and in the rest of their lives, especially at home.

At the same time, I know ordinary men who lead humble lives and yet are superpotent from head to toe. I hope that all men and women will come to see that penis power does not derive from owning mansions, yachts, and jewels or by driving Bentleys and buying expensive bottles of champagne at nightclubs. Penis power emanates from the heart and soul of a man. It is far more valuable than the costliest luxury. In a word, it is priceless.

The Character of the Superpotent Man

Penis power is about *inner qualities* That is why the most im portant point to take away from this discussion is that you are in control of your penis and your sexual destiny. What follows are the primary characteristics of superpotent men. They are within the reach of every man. As you read the following descriptions, ask yourself to what extent you possess these traits. If you find that you lack strength in a particular area, make it a personal goal to develop those traits as part of your efforts to maximize your penis power and, ultimately, your happiness.

The Superpotent Man Exudes Self-Confidence

Self-confidence is one of the most important qualities of a superpotent man. To be a man of penis power, you must believe in yourself. You must feel that you can accomplish whatever you put your mind to. Superpotent men know who they are emotionally and spiritually. They accept what they are physically but work hard to change what they can. They feel good about themselves and their place in the world. They have a certain contentment you do not see in the men who are afflicted with self-doubt. At the same time, they do not rest on their laurels. They are always working toward new goals. They are curious about life and interested in exploring new opportunities. They thrive on new challenges and new adventures. They pursue their interests and ambitions with a boundless passion and zeal.

The Superpotent Man Expresses His Full Potential

I often ask men, "What are the things you've never done but want to do?" I have noticed that superpotent men often have to think for a good while before they answer. They might mention a few seemingly inconsequential items, such as the adventurous trip they have not yet been able to take or an ambitious task like "writing that novel" they have not had time to write. But they answer with a distinct lack of concern, as if they know it will all get done in time. This is very different from the urgency and remorse expressed by men with major unfulfilled desires. Superpotent men do not look back on their lives with regret. For the most part, they have achieved the goals they set for themselves at a particular stage of their lives. These men achieve success because they live up to their potential in every respect of their work, in their relationships, and with themselves.

A colleague of mine, a fellow of enormous penis power in my estimation, captured this attitude best when we were on an exciting ski trip together. While riding up a ski lift, I asked him if there were things he had never done and wanted to do. The air was incredibly crisp and rejuvenating, and the sky was a perfectly crystal blue. My friend surveyed the glorious scene, reflecting in silence, and finally responded by saying, "There are some things I'd still like to do. But if I were to die today, I would have no regrets." Superpotent men succeed because they exercise their full potential at every moment of their lives.

The Superpotent Man Is a Winner

If you have been following the characteristics of a superpotent man, then you can see why the superpotent man *is* a winner. Not only is he hardworking and passionate, but he also believes in himself and always gives 110 percent. He puts his heart and soul into all pursuits. Men with penis power tend to enjoy competition in a healthy way. Of course, they like to come in first, but they are good sports when they lose because they know they have done their best. Their self-worth does not hinge on being number one every time. Superpotent men are successful in overcoming challenges because even though they work hard to achieve a set goal, they still enjoy the sheer exhilaration of the pursuit itself. They understand that a satisfying experience can be just as important as a favorable outcome. To these men, what truly matters is that they always try their best. When things go wrong, superpotent men bounce back quickly. Superpotent men do not think of setbacks as failures. They see them as motivation to forge ahead with an even greater degree of confidence. These men assess their actions with honesty and clarity. They learn from their mistakes and pick up the pieces with fresh determination.

The characteristics of winners are not superhuman qualities and are not contingent on any extraordinary physical or mental skill.

These qualities reflect the emotional and psychological poise of successful individuals—a success that any hardworking and determined individual can achieve.

The Superpotent Man Is Courageous

You want the superpotent man on your side when the going gets tough. He thrives under pressure. He keeps his cool, and he does not hesitate to take charge in a crisis. Whether or not he is a leader in the classic sense of the word is unimportant. What is important is that he adopts the *attitude* of a leader. He might not be in a position of authority, but when situations get tough, he is the kind of person who knows how to convert fear and tension into positive motivation and effective action. Superpotent men have the courage to face difficult challenges. They have the confidence to assume responsibility even when others are in charge.

The Superpotent Man Is Happy

If there were a motto for superpotency, it would probably be "Enjoy life to the fullest and the rest will follow." Whatever you do, wherever you are, if you are not completely aware and involved, then you are not living up to your fullest potential, and neither will your penis.

Take advantage of the present moment for all it's worth. Most of all, learn to extract the positive aspects from every situation. Penis power and a good sense of humor go hand in hand. Not that you have to be as funny as Robin Williams or have a sparkling wit that lights up a room, but you should have a certain twinkle in your eye that says, "I do not take myself *or* my life too seriously." You might be quiet and reserved or outgoing and extroverted. Whatever your personality might be, do not let fear, anxiety, nervousness, or any other weakening emotions take away your happiness. If you learn to appreciate the ironies and absurdities of life, you can laugh just as exuberantly at your own foibles as you do at a good joke.

If life throws a tragedy at you, it is appropriate to be sad. It is acceptable to be vulnerable and to be affected by loss and grief. But if you want to be a man of penis power, you cannot allow tragedy to defeat your spirit. You cannot grow bitter at the world by allowing yourself to feel like a victim. Understanding your emotions and learning how to handle the ups and downs of life is not only necessary for your own emotional health and spiritual well-being, but it is also a crucial part of developing a healthy connection between your mind, sexuality, and penis.

The Superpotent Man Is Well-Rounded

Unlike one-dimensional men, superpotent men derive pleasure from many aspects of their lives. They approach every activity with a sense of excitement, enthusiasm, and appreciation. They are able to fashion all of the positive characteristics we have discussed into one cohesive and functioning reality. This usually translates to having a wide range of interests, hobbies, and pursuits. Whether it is community service, a local sports club, fishing, arts, chess, golf, or wining and dining, superpotent men have an expansive interest in life.

They love to learn about new things, try new foods, and explore new countries. They allow their personalities to benefit from the education they receive. Becoming superpotent does not mean you have to become involved in countless meaningless activities. What I mean by "well-rounded" is having a continuous interest in expanding your personality and knowledge. The only way to broaden your horizons and keep your life exciting is to avoid any kind of stagnant monotony throughout your years—a monotony that can be especially detrimental to penis power.

The Superpotent Man Has Quality Relationships

Superpotent men work hard to have quality relationships in both their business and personal lives. A psychiatrist friend once told me that strong, successful men know that they *need* other people. They respect the roles that other people play in their lives, and they understand that they cannot achieve their goals alone. Weak individuals who are selfish and ungrateful *use* other people in a degrading and unhealthy way, usually in an attempt to feel powerful. Superpotent men treat people with respect and, therefore, command the same from others. They possess a certain charm and ease in social situations because they are sensitive to the feelings of others. Superpotent men take advantage of kindness and generosity. They show respect and consideration as ways to build healthy and strong relationships with the people in their lives.

The Superpotent Man and Sex

The qualities we've discussed are the general qualities of superpotent men. These qualities are all readily attainable if you are willing to adjust your beliefs and attitude. If you have the courage to recognize areas in your life that need work, and if you have the strength to make the appropriate changes, you will undoubtedly see huge improvements in your self-image, your interpersonal relationships, and in every other area of your life.

In the following section, we will look specifically at the attitudes and behaviors of the Superpotent Man as they pertain to sex.

Keep in mind that personality and penis traits are fundamentally connected. If you are someone who desires to become not only a great person but also a great lover, you must be willing to confront yourself and address the aspects of your personality that may be holding you back from emotional and sexual happiness.

If you and your partner are having relationship problems because of personality or behavioral habits, it is important to have an open and honest discussion about the real issues involved. Using this book as a reference guide is a great way to break the ice and make progress in your relationship.

The Superpotent Man Has a Symbiotic Relationship with His Penis

View your penis as an integral part of your physical self and your emotional self. In a certain sense, your penis is your most vital organ. Not vital in the same sense that your heart, lungs, and kidneys are vital—that is, if they do not function properly you die—but vital in the sense that your penis is the organ that expresses your spirit and individuality.

The superpotent man has a positive penis image to go along with his positive self-image. He loves his penis. He respects it. He treats it well. He takes care of it and never worries about it.

Take pride in your penis. It is your friend and partner in the pursuit of happiness.

Let me distinguish the man of penis power from the others who might *seem* to have those characteristics. The superpotent man is not obsessed with his penis. He is not dominated by it. Obsession is a sign of penis weakness. If you meet a man who is obviously penis obsessed—a guy who is led around by his penis like a slave—he is most likely not a superpotent man. He is probably disconnected from his penis or in conflict with it. He is to be pitied, not admired. Men who are really in control of their lives and their sexualities—men with penis power—usually do not *seem* to be penis oriented. There is a powerful nonchalance to their style. Carry your penis pride with dignity. You have nothing to prove, and you have nothing to hide.

It is also important to realize that *superpotency has nothing to do with the size or appearance of your penis.* The man who has penis power does not have some golden rod or magic wand hanging between his legs. As an experienced urologist, I can assure you that the penis of a superpotent man has no special attributes that separate it from the penises of the rest of the species. The differences are all in the mind.

The Superpotent Man Has a High Level of Penis Awareness

He who understands his penis knows himself. It may sound like a cliché, but it could not be more true. Make an effort to learn about the anatomy and physiology of your penis. Get in touch with the likes and dislikes and quirks and foibles of your own individual penis. Ultimately, your mind and your penis are controlled by the same axis. When you are tired or upset, your penis will behave differently than when you are energetic and upbeat. If you are angry with your partner, your penis will express that feeling, too. If you adore your partner, there is no doubt that the attitude of your penis will show it.

Penis awareness creates a smooth and harmonious functioning between your mind and your penis. The superpotent penis will do what its owner expects it to do. If you develop a healthy relationship with the emotions in your mind, your penis will conduct itself in a manner consistent with how you want it to behave. Like a trustworthy business partner, your penis is far less likely to disappoint you or come up with unpleasant surprises.

The Superpotent Man Has an Extremely Satisfying Sex Life

If statistics were taken, superpotent men would be way above average in terms of frequency of sex and quality of performance. This is not because they have gifted penises, but because they have a positive penis attitude. This will be true whether you are a single man with a variety of sex partners or a monogamous man with one partner for life. It will be true whether you are young and handsome or aging and ordinary.

It is important to dispel any notion that penis power is about performing Olympian sexual feats. Superpotent men do not go out and break records for frequency of intercourse, the number of orgasms their partners have, or the number of times they can achieve an erection in a night. Those are not the criteria for penis power. If they were, then the men who perform in pornographic films would be the epitome of penis power because they can accomplish incredible sexual feats. They get erect on command and ejaculate whenever the director orders it. But porn stars are not men of penis power.

In my practice, I have had many male pornographic film stars as patients. I would not categorize a single one of them as a superpotent man. They represent an inflated, overeroticized concept of male sexual power—an image that should not be viewed as having any relation to true penis power.

Do not measure your sexual self-worth by performance criteria.

Any man whose self-image hinges on superficial things like how often he scores and how great he performs does *not* meet the standards of true penis power. To be a superpotent man, you must view sex as an intimate pleasure, not as a sporting event. Sex is not show business. You are not there to prove anything or to perform for anyone. You do not have to be what people would call a "stud." You certainly do not have to be a Don Juan or a braggart.

What should matter to you is that you use your penis as often and in such a manner as is most satisfying to both you and your partner. What you should really care about is that, when you call upon your penis, it functions according to your personal standards and not by some imaginary yardstick.

To be a man of penis power is to be content with yourself and your penis. That is the best and only criterion for satisfaction. That is not to say that the penis of a superpotent man always performs to maximum capacity. Because his penis functions in harmony with the rest of his mind and body, its success rate is much higher than the penises of most men. When the man of penis power is let down by his penis, as happens on occasion, he takes it in stride. You should understand that *such occurrences happen to all men* and are to be expected from time to time. Nine times out of ten, the causes are circumstantial and not systemic. As a superpotent man, you can be idealistic about your potential, but it is also wise to be realistic.

If you do have a disappointment, do not view it as a disaster. Do not take it as a personal failure or a sign of pathology. Do not let it affect your confidence or self-image. What others see as a problem, the man of penis power might see as a joke. He might find it terribly amusing that he and his penis are temporarily out of sync. He might see it as an opportunity to face another "penis challenge." Learn from your experience and move ahead to the next sexual opportunity without hesitation or apprehension.

The Superpotent Man Enjoys Giving and Receiving Pleasure

The superpotent man enjoys giving pleasure. Not only does he have sex often, but he also savors each and every experience. That is one of the main reasons he has sex. You should take sex seriously, not somberly. Be passionate and intense during sex. Be frivolous, whimsical, and funny if the occasion calls for it. It is okay to laugh during sex, even at yourself. The superpotent man enjoys spontaneity and unpredictability. He appreciates imaginative partners.

Most men of penis power have a wholesome appetite for new experiences. They thrive on variety. That may mean frequent encounters with an assortment of partners, or it may mean a wide spectrum of adventures with one partner. This attitude of penis power is epitomized by the riddle:

> What is the difference between sex and wrestling?
> Answer: In wrestling, some holds are barred.

Superpotent men are not womanizers or "players" in the pejorative sense of the word. Even those who avoid long-term relationships and who move from bed to bed pursue their pleasure responsibly. They exude the style and integrity of a gentleman. Penis power, as with all types of power, carries with it moral obligations. Penis power can be used to exploit and abuse, or it can be applied with generosity and sensitivity to foster healthy, meaningful relationships. Superpotent men might enjoy sex whenever and wherever they may find it, but they are not promiscuous. You do not have to pursue pleasure at the expense of a balanced life or at the cost of hurting other people's feelings. Your goal should be mutual enjoyment, not sexual conquest.

Do not succumb to what is euphemistically labeled the "hard dick syndrome" (i.e., "If my dick is harder than it has been in years, it must be true love!"). The key is to keep your wits about you even when your penis is aroused and threatening to run amok. Do not jeopardize a healthy, established relationship with a cherished partner if you are aroused in an unexpected encounter.

Do not disregard important values such as trust, honesty, consideration, and sensitivity for the sake of an orgasm. Be confident enough to know that there is always tomorrow—just like an experienced commuter does not risk his life by running wildly down the track to catch a train because he knows another will come shortly. Men of penis power are uninhibited and adventurous, but they are aware of the ramifications of their actions.

Superpotent men *do not take foolish risks*. As a urologist who has watched patients waste away and die of HIV/AIDS, I must urge you to educate yourself about sexually transmitted diseases and value your life enough to exercise your penis power prudently. You do not need to be overly cautious or terrorized to the point of paranoia (something I have seen among many heterosexual and homosexual men), but you must know the facts and learn how to enjoy an active sex life without fear. (See more on this important subject in chapter 10, "Sexually Transmitted Diseases.")

The Superpotent Man Is at Ease with His Sexuality

The superpotent man loves sex. He thinks about it often. It is important to him. That is why he enjoys it to the fullest. For most men, this attitude translates into excellent sexual performance. When the man of penis power does have a good experience, he remains humble. Men of genuine talent and ability let their achievements speak for themselves. Men who find it necessary to boast are usually compensating for some perceived weakness. Men who talk endlessly about their sex lives remind me of the target of the following joke: after examining a patient and listening to his extravagant boasts, a doctor tells him to give up half his sex life. "Which half" his wife asks, "talking about it or thinking about it?"

The man of penis power appreciates the human form in all of its shapes and sizes: the shape of a leg, the curve of a hip, and the swelling arc of a full bosom or buttock. Is there anything wrong with that? Is it exploitive or demeaning? Is it sexist or chauvinistic? No, it is natural and healthy. Despite the rhetoric of extremists, most people understand and appreciate that the human form is designed to arouse sexual interest.

We want to be attractive to other people. That is why women wear short skirts and tight pants. That is why they fuss with their hair and makeup, analyze the contours of their bust line, and shop for bras with the most seductive lift.

This is the same reason why men dress in style or wear tightly fitted clothes that accentuate their physique. It is a fact of life that people want to check out other people, and they want to be checked out, too. Men do it to women when they look them up and down or point out a real "looker" to their buddies.

Women do the same thing to men when they look at "hotties" and mentally undress them. This human urge is all part of nature's plan for keeping the species alive. We ought to acknowledge it, celebrate it, and enjoy it. Take the guilt out of sexual attraction!

We have to accept the fact that men are voyeurs and naturally act as sexual predators. But women in today's world are really no different. Let me make an important point: on some level, superpotent men view their partners as sex objects, but not as mere sex objects.

They may not admit it, but deep in the dark corners of their psyche, all men see their partners as the means to a very definitive sexual end. Women see men as sex objects as well. Problems arise when men treat their partners as if all they are good for is ogling or pawing or to provide a moist, warm place to put their penises.

The real troubles in sexual relationships arise when men fail to relate to their partners as complete human beings. Superpotent men do not have this problem. They appreciate all dimensions of their lovers. They have no need to feel superior. They are at ease in the company of their partners, and the feeling is mutual.

The superpotent man loves sex, and he loves to chase after sexual opportunities. A superpotent man pursues a liaison with a certain degree of persistence. It is important to acknowledge the fine line in the delicate dance of sex, though. The superpotent man always behaves with sensitivity, awareness, and integrity. He knows where to draw the line, especially when a partner says no! All men must be made aware that respecting boundaries is a very significant topic among women today.

Do not infer any conclusion from a partner's body language. Forcing a sex partner into doing something he does not want to do is absolutely unacceptable.

Superpotent men understand that rejection is a function of circumstances and individual taste, rather than a personal affront. Therefore, these men have no need to force themselves on anyone, and they have no desire to hurt anyone. They have judgment. As a surgeon, I often say you can teach a gorilla how to do an appendectomy, but you cannot teach a gorilla when to do one. That takes judgment, and in sexual behavior, as in surgery, judgment separates the men from the boys. Men of true penis power do not use lies or deception to manipulate someone into bed. They certainly do not use physical force. They do not play games that can cause anyone pain or anguish. The superpotent man is a man of incredible sensitivity and consideration. Those qualities always work to his advantage.

The Superpotent Man Gives Openly and without Reservation

You should care about your partner's sexual pleasure as much as your own. You should do this not for the sake of macho pride or because you are a self-sacrificing saint. You should care because you value your partner's satisfaction. In addition, you know that the more you give, the more you will receive in return.

Superpotent men understand the sensitive nature of feelings and the importance of open and honest communication. Listen when your partner tells you she likes or dislikes what you are doing. Do your best to accommodate her preferences. Sometimes these clues may not be as obvious as your partner shouting out "Yes!" but rather they may come in the form of body language or a heightened reaction.

Pay attention to the subtle clues your partner may be giving you. Feel free to *ask* him if what you are doing is good or bad. Talking about sex while it is happening is not only a huge turnon for a lot of people, it is also a guaranteed way of finding the right moves to satisfy your partner. The same goes for expressing your own needs and preferences. You should have no reservations about asking your partner to do the things that you desire.

The Superpotent Man Does Not Have Performance Anxiety

Perhaps the most salient distinction between men with penis power and men with penis weakness is the presence or absence of performance anxiety. Several studies have been done in which sex partners have been observed in very aroused states, usually brought on by the viewing of erotic videos.

The men who had stated earlier that they performed in a satisfactory manner showed a marked increase in arousal after viewing the erotic films. This was in sharp contrast with the men who had admitted some degree of sexual dysfunction. That group had a marked *decrease* in arousal after watching the movies. Why? Because as their partners became more responsive, they started concentrating on performance concerns and the anxieties they associated with sex. They worried whether they would function well. The other, more confident men focused on the erotic cues of their aroused partners and got even more turned on.

This is exactly why, as a superpotent man, you will be able to give your partner greater satisfaction. You will not be inhibited by self-doubt. You will respond to your partner's arousal with the full confidence that you will "rise" to the occasion.

Men of penis power develop a positive feedback loop. It starts with an aroused partner or an invitation to sex. This immediately registers a positive expectation of the forthcoming experience. It is followed by an accurate assessment of the sexual demand that is being made and a direct focus on meeting the demand with a radar-like ability to tune into a partner's cues. Men of penis power do not focus on their own fears about performance. They focus on the wonderful experience they are about to share. This simple shift in mind-frame automatically leads to greater penis arousal. This arousal loops around to a heightened attention to sexual cues. What results is a mutually satisfying sexual experience and an increase in confidence.

By contrast, men of penis weakness have a negative feedback loop. A sexual proposition elicits a negative expectation. This leads to self-consciousness. Self-consciousness leads to an inability to perceive a partner's cues, which leads to decreased arousal. This path confirms negative expectations, increasing performance anxiety. This anxiety prevents adequate performance. All of this leads to future avoidance of sex and future failure.

To become a man of penis power, you must become a master of the positive sexual feedback loop. Otherwise, negativity and performance anxiety will lessen your sexual potential.

The Superpotent Man Knows How to Handle Stress

Superpotent men do not succumb to the debilitating power of anxiety or depression. Superpotent men often find themselves in relationships that other men may find inhibiting, such as having an aggressive partner or being with someone who may prefer unusual sexual practices.

To a man with penis weakness, these might be stressful situations that elicit fear and self-doubt. The superpotent man responds like an athlete who is up against a worthy opponent or who has teamed up with a great partner. Such a situation brings out the best in him.

The superpotent attitude is "My penis is my friend. What's good for him is good for me. He never lets me down." If you start to feel anxious, turn that feeling into positive energy. You can convert that edginess into stimulation and become even *more* aroused.

Nothing is more debilitating to sexual satisfaction than anxiety and depression. Even though depression is known to diminish sexual desire and responsiveness, this result is not inevitable. The emotional contours of a man's life do not have to interfere with his sexuality. Even a superpotent man is vulnerable to the occasional situational depression. Every man is vulnerable to the worries and fears that afflict all people at one time or another. If you have faith in yourself, develop a healthy method for dealing with your emotions, and learn how to extract the positive elements from every experience, you will climb out of depressions quickly and convert your worries into effective action.

To become a man of penis power, you must develop the capacity to prevent negative emotions from impeding your ability to achieve an erection. You cannot let the stress of your outside life intrude into the bedroom. If you are depressed, rest assured that your penis will also be depressed.

Penis Power Is Defined by Who You Are and How You Control Your Life

You should now have a clear understanding of the chief characteristics of superpotent men. Superpotent men are not all shaped by the same cookie cutter. They share the majority of these important behavioral and attitudinal patterns, but there is a tremendous range of variation among men with penis power. They are tall and short, plain and handsome, young and old, rich and poor. Their penises are big, small, and average. They have sex all the time, frequently, or just occasionally. They are bold and aggressive or coy and self-effacing. They like women who are blonde, brunette, or redheaded, dark or pale, tall or short, buxom or slim. During sex they prefer the missionary position, sitting up, or the canine way, or with their partner on top—or all of the above. They like sex in the morning, at night, in the afternoon, or at all times of day.

Discovering your penis power does not come from imitating someone else or from living up to a hypothetical standard set by an external source. It comes from examining the aspects of your personality, relationships, and self-image that you want to improve and from making those needed changes. Penis power is about self-understanding and self-expression. Most of all, it is about realizing your full potential. There are an infinite number of ways to express penis power. Your way is as good as anyone else's way. The important thing is to harness that power and use it to extract the most pleasure from your entire life.

Superpotency is within the reach of every man. It is not a super-human state. It is normal and natural. You will be surprised how easy it is to achieve. Self-doubt, and the penis weakness it creates, is a *temporary* sickness that can only be cured by your own will-power. I have seen men become superpotent after learning a few facts and getting a simple pep talk from me. They readjust their attitudes about themselves and their penises. They adopt positive personality traits and reject the old, negative traits that were hold-ing them back. After that, they're off and running with great re-sults almost immediately. Other men have to work at it for some time or must use the specific procedures you will find in this book. These tips have helped men change their sexual behavior, giving them added penis power and serving as proof to themselves and their partners that they are capable of being superpotent.

The sixty-four-dollar question is, "How do I become a superpo-tent man?" The following chapter will give you (and your partner) all the answers.

Chapter 15

How to Become a Superpotent Man

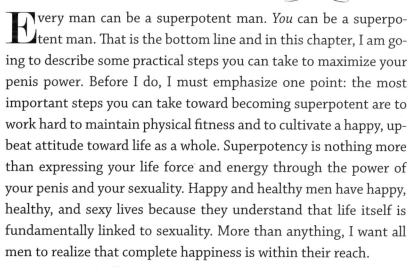

Every man can be a superpotent man. *You* can be a superpotent man. That is the bottom line and in this chapter, I am going to describe some practical steps you can take to maximize your penis power. Before I do, I must emphasize one point: the most important steps you can take toward becoming superpotent are to work hard to maintain physical fitness and to cultivate a happy, upbeat attitude toward life as a whole. Superpotency is nothing more than expressing your life force and energy through the power of your penis and your sexuality. Happy and healthy men have happy, healthy, and sexy lives because they understand that life itself is fundamentally linked to sexuality. More than anything, I want all men to realize that complete happiness is within their reach.

More specifically, you should develop in yourself the positive qualities of a superpotent man (see chapter 13). If you emulate these as closely as possible and shape your behavior and attitude accordingly, increasing your penis power will be an easy and effective task.

Educate Yourself

I am constantly amazed by men's relative ignorance about sexuality in general and women in particular. I have known men with highly sophisticated minds, wide-ranging experience, and excellent educations who fit this profile. They do not know a clitoris from a cuticle, and it is not because they are not interested in sex. On the contrary, they are *very* interested in sex. They complain that they cannot "figure women out." The problem is magnified because they do not educate themselves. Their disconnect comes from being overly interested in their own satisfaction and not interested enough in their partners'.

This is the wrong attitude for a superpotent penis-power man. Part of becoming superpotent involves caring a great deal about satisfying your partner's needs and desires, not just for reasons of equality and generosity but also out of pure *self-interest*. I am not certain about the rest of life, but in sex you really do reap what you sow. It is truly better to give more to your partner than you receive because, in the long run, nothing excites a penis more than a wildly responsive lover. Satisfy your lover, and she will react by finding ways to please you in a manner you never thought possible.

We know that women are different from men, but a heterosexual man of penis power should understand *exactly how* women are different. This is not the place for a treatise on this subject. Many books are devoted entirely to women's sexuality—a subject in which I believe all men should be experts. That being said, I would like to single out one point that many men do not fully appreciate. For physiological reasons, women generally take longer than men to get aroused. As one of my patients observed, "Women are like radio tubes—it takes them time to warm up. Men are like transistors—solid-state and turned on instantly." For this reason, women often complain that men denigrate foreplay, and men complain that women want to fool around too much before "getting down to business."

Each partner must learn to accommodate the other. If sometimes a man is so turned on that he has no time for the niceties of foreplay, his partner should try to understand this particularly urgent expression of passion. All men, regardless of their passionate urges, must learn to appreciate a partner's desire for the subtle and sensual pleasures of foreplay and learn to satisfy this need with patience and generosity. Technically speaking, foreplay is necessary to lubricate a woman's vagina, which helps prevent sex from being painful or irritating. If you are impatient with foreplay, you might be missing out on some of life's sweetest pleasures. You are also depriving yourself of the great satisfaction that comes from giving pleasure to your partner. Men who learn to satisfy their lovers' needs prior to intercourse find that their penis power increases measurably.

Even more important than understanding women's sexuality in general is learning about your specific partner's sexuality. There is tremendous variation among women. They have a vast range of likes and dislikes. You should never assume that the woman you are with fits a stereotype or has the same sexual preferences as your past partners. Honest and open one-on-one communication is essential. Many men are uncomfortable talking about sex with women, even the ones they have been with for years. If you want to be a superpotent man, break the ice. Find out what pleases your woman or partner most. Find out what he really desires, what he fantasizes about, what he wants you to do more of or less of. A partner who is open and honest is one of the best allies a penis can have.

Equally important is a partner who is responsive to *your* needs. It is amazing how many men complain to *me* that their lovers do not do enough of this or do too much of that when they never even bother to discuss it with *them*. You should be up front about your preferences. Communicate in a caring way without any unnecessary pressure, criticism, or ultimatums. If she is willing to make the effort, it will surely enhance your penis power. If she is *not* willing to make the effort, then you might be in a sexually incompatible relationship, or you might have to sort out some of the deeper reasons for her resistance. Unless your desires run to dangerous sex or your partner has personal limitations and boundaries, you deserve to have your wishes met; in turn, you also must be willing to meet your partner halfway.

A final word to those learning about sex: do not overdo it. If you overintellectualize, you may create an impediment. You can get so bogged down with facts and diagrams and psychological theories that you end up being even more self-conscious and inhibited than when you first started. If you end up thinking too much, you may lose the spontaneity and passion that makes sex so wonderful. I say: if you overanalyze it, you paralyze it. If you subject your sexuality to overintellectualization, your penis will be saying, "Wake me up when you stop thinking so much."

Good Health Equals Good Penis Power

The general condition of your mind and body is reflected in the health of your penis power. For that reason, it is vital for superpotent men to maintain a high level of well-being, both mentally and physically. Here are some basic tips.

Get Fit and Stay Fit

A good exercise program is central to overall health and sexual fitness. It takes energy and strength to make love. The muscles of your arms, legs, back, and abdomen are all involved. If they become flabby, your penis also risks becoming flabby. Build up your muscular strength with weights, push-ups, sit-ups, yoga, or whatever exercise you prefer. It is not that you have to be "ripped" or sculpted like a Greek god, but it is important to develop muscular strength and flexibility.

Commit to Cardiovascular Fitness

A vigorous half hour of aerobic exercises four or five times a week is what I recommend for developing and maintaining cardiovascular fitness. Physical inactivity leads to deterioration of your body as a whole and can also lead to deterioration of your penis power. If you start wheezing or gasping for breath while making love, your penis will get the message that you need to rest, and that is exactly what it will do.

Pay Attention to What You Eat

A diet low in saturated fat and high in fiber is the most effective diet for maintaining penis power. We have discussed the importance of blood flow in getting and keeping an erection. It is obvious that superpotency depends on clean arteries. Do not gum up the works by ingesting saturated fats and bad cholesterol. If you have ever made love when you felt bloated or constipated, you know how much better you function when your digestive system is not overtaxed. Do not overeat; make sure you consume plenty of fiber. Wining and dining can be romantic, but the romance withers if you overdo either one. Too much alcohol (or any intoxicant) might increase your desire, but will surely diminish your penis power. Too much dining, and you will feel sluggish, heavy, and tired. In addition, a superpotent man should be concerned with maintaining good prostate health. Reliable evidence supports a low-fat, high-fiber, and high-protein diet in addition to regular exercise as part of a good overall regimen to keep your prostate healthy.

Maintain Weight Control

Let us face it—it is a lot easier to operate smoothly and vigorously in bed if you are not carrying a twenty-pound belt of blubber around your waist. Not only are there health risks to being overweight, but for most women, a lean physique is much more attractive. Even more important than how other people see you is *your* perception of your body. Maintaining a healthy body weight encourages self-confidence and promotes a healthy and positive outlook on life. In addition, if you are overweight and looking down at your penis from above a big belly, you might start thinking of your penis as small because layers of fat obscure so much of it. That, in turn, will cause you to *think* small about your penis power.

In general, I have found that men with poor body images have some degree of penis weakness. Men who are comfortable with their bodies and are content with their looks have a higher likelihood for superpotency. Believe it or not, men with positive body images are not necessarily hunks. Some good-looking, well-built men have far *worse* body images than men with ordinary bodies. It is all a matter of how you see yourself. Some men are so insecure and vain that if they do not see Brad Pitt when they look in the mirror, they hate their bodies and ultimately spread a pall of negativity on their self-esteem. Others are content with what nature gave them as long as they stay in reasonable shape. In my opinion, every man is capable of realizing his personal body image goals. To start, set your own standards of health and fitness and maintain a regular routine.

Do Not Hold Your Penis Power Hostage to the Youth Cult Perpetuated by the Media

Those images of sleek, muscular bodies with gorgeous women at their sides promoting everything from deodorant to pickup trucks are detrimental to superpotency. Whose self-image could possibly live up to those standards? Avoid comparing yourself to other men, especially images of men in magazines and in movies. If you eat right, exercise regularly, and maintain a sensible weight, you will feel good about your body and yourself as a whole. If you feel good about your body, you will feel good about the appendage that represents your sexual power—your penis.

Get Plenty of Rest

Superpotent men tend to live balanced lives. They are energetic, busy, and productive, but they are not workaholics in the obsessive sense of the word. In my experience, many workaholics seem to be running away from something. If they drown themselves in work just to make up for some deep feeling of inadequacy, they often jeopardize good relationships with their partners. Superpotent men, on the other hand, are usually just as *productive* as workaholics and they work just as hard, but they also work *intelligently*. They know when and how to relax. Their capacity for fun is as big as their capacity for work. They have that seemingly uncanny ability to compartmentalize their lives.

Maintain Good Mental Health

In addition to good physical health, penis power requires sound mental health. I have already discussed the need to reduce stress, tension, anxiety, depression, and other enemies of penis power. It bears repeating here: stress will weaken you physically, interfere with the biochemical action needed to produce erections, and possibly lower your self-image to the point where you doubt your manhood.

Numerous studies have shown that people who undergo major traumas, such as the loss of a loved one or an accident, are much more likely to experience a serious illness. I can add unequivocally that they are more likely to exhibit penis weakness as well. I have seen many patients suffering from post-traumatic stress syndrome, and I can tell you that their penises often behave just like the men themselves: confused, frightened, and helpless. With my superpotent patients, however, even serious traumas do not seem to have such a devastating effect. These individuals appear to deal with a crisis in a healthy, effective way. When the crisis resolves, they put it behind them, and their stressful encounter fades quickly from their minds. If you do not learn to deal with life's difficulties in a positive way, traumas large and small will pollute all aspects of your life, especially your penis power. It takes strength, confidence, and self-awareness to be a superpotent man. It is these very qualities that are needed to overcome stressful situations.

Penis Power Exercises

One particular form of exercise is the best way to develop penis power: *sex*! Practice makes perfect in bed, just as it does in a sports stadium or concert hall. The more you use your penis and the more you learn about using it, the more control you will gain over its functioning.

Making love is a great form of exercise for your whole body. Vigorous sex increases the volume of oxygen in your lungs, quickens your heart rate, and raises your effective circulating blood volume, all of which benefit your general health. Sex can also help you moderate potentially dangerous habits. When you are sexually satisfied, you feel so good about yourself that you are less likely to abuse drugs, alcohol, or junk food. Finally, sex is a great antidote for stress (if not the greatest!). If you are feeling anxious or worried, if you need to steer your mind away from burdensome thoughts and work off some tension, then having sex is the best solution.

Just as there are specific exercises to help you improve in a sport, there are ways to improve your penis power by strengthening the muscles used during sex. There is no sense in exercising the penis itself because, physically speaking, it is a passive organ without any muscles. However, you *can* exercise other body parts that serve the penis during sex. This strengthening will give you greater control of your movements, as well as added stamina, vigor, and flexibility. You are also likely to notice an increase of confidence in your penis power.

One suggestion is to do push-ups or weight exercises that use the same basic motion of pushing and pulling with the upper arms and chest muscles. To the extent that you support your body with your arms while making love, this conditioning will help prevent fatigue, so that your penis will not be thinking, "Hurry up and get it over with!" Squats, knee bends, or other exercises for the upper legs, as well as exercises that strengthen the abdominal muscles, will all increase penis power because those muscles help support you during various sexual positions.

Maybe Elvis Was on to Something: Pelvic Control

One of the most important areas in which to develop strength is the pelvic region. If you have control of your pelvis, your penis will function more creatively and dynamically. To accomplish this, I strongly suggest working on the muscles of the abdomen and lower back. Sit-ups, crunches, leg raises, and similar exercises will help a great deal. More to the point, I advise working on the flexibility of the pelvic region itself.

A colleague of mine, Lucien Martin, who is a chiropractor in Santa Monica, California, has developed a more systematic form of pelvic exercise. Dr. Martin created a series of exercises to strengthen the muscles of the lower back and abdomen for patients with back problems. To his surprise, his patients reported dramatic improvements in their sex lives. He developed the exercises further and continued to get the same reports. According to Dr. Martin, the exercises strengthen the muscles and ligaments of the pelvis, lower back, and abdomen, and they seem to improve nerve sensitivity in that area. Here are Dr. Martin's instructions for his pelvic control technique.

> Lie on your back on the floor or on a very firm bed, arms at your sides. Place a tightly rolled towel of three to four inches in diameter under your neck, not your head. Place a thick pillow under your knees so that your lower back rests flat on the floor. Now, without

Becoming a Superpotent Man

lifting your lower back off the floor, pull your pubic bone toward your chest. Do not suck in your stomach. The idea is to lift the pelvis by *squeezing* the abdominal muscles like an accordion, not to pull them inward.

Lock the pelvis in the compressed position for about a second and then relax. Then repeat the same pattern again and again. To make sure you are doing it correctly, press your lower abdominal muscles with the fingers of both hands as you do the squeeze. You should feel those core muscles contract. Another way to test yourself is to press the abdominal muscles while raising your head and legs slightly. You should feel the compression of the muscles used during the exercise.

Proper breathing during the exercise is very important. Keep your throat and mouth relaxed. As you squeeze your abdominals, let the motion of your pelvis expel the air from your lungs. Do not breathe out forcefully, and do not hold your breath. Exhale smoothly as you contract your abdominals, and inhale smoothly as you relax.

The exercise should be brief and vigorous. Hold each contraction for about a second and continue the repetitions for two to three minutes. Once you gain good control, you can set a goal of one hundred repetitions per day. One note of caution: if you have acute lower back problems, do not undertake this exercise without first consulting your orthopedist.

The Harder They Come: Controlling Your Timing

Superpotency is not only about getting an erection at the right time, it also involves controlling the timing of your orgasm to provide maximum satisfaction for you and your partner. As mentioned in chapter 4, problems with ejaculation come in two basic categories: too fast and too slow.

The latter of the two is called retarded ejaculation and can be caused by medical factors such as spinal cord injury or diabetes, as well as by substance abuse or the side effects of certain medications. In rare instances, the problem is so extreme that a man may be unable to ejaculate at all. Obviously, this requires the attention of a urologist. In other cases, the problem is psychological in origin. Some men can masturbate to climax *and* even have nocturnal emissions (spontaneous ejaculation at night), but cannot ejaculate in a vagina or with their partners. This is usually rooted in self-doubt, repressed trauma, fear of pregnancy, or anxiety over committing to a relationship. These types of psychological problems can be dealt with best by psychological counseling.

By far, the most common reason for retarded ejaculation is the normal aging process. As mentioned earlier, men who develop problems controlling their ejaculate might come to view this issue as a positive development because sex lasts longer and both partners are more satisfied. But this can be problematic, especially in an older couple exhausting themselves by pumping away furiously to induce an orgasm while the vagina becomes irritated. For an older couple, patience and a little creativity (i.e., lubrication) are usually enough to solve the problem. I suggest you vary your positions and avoid any particularly strenuous sexual activities. Build up gradually, using less violent forms of stimulation. Do not hesitate to stop and rest when you need to do so. Experiment with various oils and lotions; the lubrication just might increase sensitivity enough to facilitate orgasm.

The more troubling problem is premature ejaculation. Those dreaded words conjure up images of humiliation, failed masculinity, and frustrated women running to their vibrators. As discussed in chapter 4, there is some degree of variation in the way the medical community defines premature ejaculation. Some sex therapists classify it as the inability to delay ejaculation for at least five minutes. Others take a more flexible approach, defining it as the inability to delay ejaculation long enough to satisfy your partner in at least half of your sexual encounters. That perspective recognizes that it is normal for the time of ejaculation to vary and for it to sometimes fall short of the ideal.

It is impossible to come up with a universal definition of premature ejaculation because there is so much variation among individuals. I have met women who are perfectly satisfied with intercourse that lasts two or three minutes, while others are frustrated when their husbands cannot last more than fifteen or twenty. It comes down to individual judgment: do you and your partner feel that you reach orgasm too quickly? If so, there are many practical steps you can take to solve the problem.

Even if you *do not* have a problem, the following suggestions are worthy of your attention. They will enhance your penis power by improving your ejaculatory control, and they will make your orgasms more intense.

First, let me make a few basic points. The most common cause of premature ejaculation is quite simply sexual inactivity. It is a matter of common sense. When the seminal vesicles are filled to capacity, it takes very little stimulation to start the ejaculatory reflex. This is because the fluid simply has to be released. This is why every man experiences quick ejaculation on occasion. It is also why it happens most often to younger men. They produce a much larger *volume* of seminal fluid, and the ejaculatory reflex is volume-related.

However, infrequent sex is not the only cause. When premature ejaculation becomes chronic, it is usually because of patterns rooted in early experience. For many young men, initial sexual encounters are not only characterized by anxiety and fear but also by time pressure. After only a few repeated experiences, what once was a little bit of anxiety and nervousness can become a chronic condition of premature ejaculation. For some young men, early experiences of sex can be a solitary pursuit. Those teenagers who masturbate in the bathroom or under their sheets can become self-conscious to the point of paranoia. With those young men, their goal is not to *delay* ejaculation, but to get it over with as quickly as possible before they are discovered.

Ultimately, these types of early experiences establish a *low threshold of excitement*. Most men who develop this low threshold become conditioned to ejaculate quickly. If they do not make a conscious effort to change that pattern, they can become chronic premature ejaculators. I have often treated young men who are so humiliated by premature ejaculation that they develop a strong sense of inadequacy and shy away from sex altogether. The problem is frequently compounded by erectile dysfunction.

Whatever the initial cause, it is important not to view early ejaculation as a personal failure. If it occasionally happens, it is probably due to a long lapse between orgasms or to nervousness: a new, passionate love affair might be so exciting that the threshold for orgasm is lowered considerably. Even if the problem is chronic, I can assure you that it is not a sign of permanent inadequacy or diminished manhood, but simply a matter of bad habits that can be changed with practice and patience.

The good news is that no matter where you start from, you can vastly increase your ejaculatory control. Using the procedures I am about to describe, I have helped patients who reached orgasm in less than two minutes improve to where they could last more than half an hour after a few weeks or months of practice.

One point is important to make in this context: if you are in an ongoing relationship, it is important to win the support of your partner. Early ejaculation can be extremely frustrating for yourself *and* your partner. If it continues for a long time, it can lead to resentment. Many women have told me that they sometimes feel that their men are not even *trying* to slow down and that they care only about their own needs. Some women say they feel used. You must convince your partner that you are sincere about improving your staying power. Tell him that you would be grateful for his patience and help. The basic goal is to delay ejaculation to a point that is most satisfying for *both* of you.

The "Tain't" Exercises

The following exercise, which is similar to that developed by gynecologist Arnold Kegel for female patients with urinary incontinence, will help give you greater control of your ejaculations and also increase the intensity of your orgasms.

Earlier, we saw that the muscles in the perineum (the "tain't")— the area between the scrotum and the anus—are involved in the ejaculatory process. If you were to put your finger in that area when you ejaculate, you would feel the contractions. If you placed a mirror between your legs, you would see the whole area contract like a flexing bicep. Anatomically, these muscles support the urinary sphincter, so they are the ones you contract when you are forced to hold in your urine or stop its flow. Try it the next time you urinate: when you stop the flow, the muscles you contract are the very ones we are talking about. By strengthening the muscles of the perineum, you will pump more blood to this vital area, achieve greater ejaculatory control, and increase the intensity of your orgasms.

The basic idea is to contract and relax the muscles repeatedly, as you would in any strengthening program. You can do this either standing up or sitting down. To do this exercise, use your mind's eye to isolate the muscle surrounding the anal sphincter. Imagine that you have inserted a rectal thermometer and are trying to pull it up into your body, right up to your Adam's apple. Do not hunch your shoulders and do not squeeze your buttocks together. The muscles involved are all internal. Squeeze them and hold that position for ten counts. Then relax and repeat the process several times.

As with any new exercise, the muscles will feel tired at first. Do not do it to exhaustion, but increase the number of repetitions until you can comfortably do one hundred during the course of a day. Do these exercises consistently and you will, in time, notice the benefits I described. Once you begin to notice improvement, I suggest that you continue to do the exercises to maintain the improvement and progress even further. You can do them anytime: while driving, walking, standing in line, or watching television. When done correctly, they are totally unobtrusive. If someone can see you doing the exercise, then you are doing it wrong.

A recent incident compels me to repeat one instruction. A patient to whom I taught these exercises came in a week later and said, "I've noticed an improvement, Doc. The exercise is working great, but my asshole is sore as hell. Sticking that thermometer up there a hundred times a day is murder!" So I repeat: *imagine* you are inserting a rectal thermometer; do not actually do it!

Techniques for Delaying Ejaculation

The key to prolonging intercourse is to become so well tuned to your own body mechanisms that you can take action to hold off ejaculation *before* it is too late. Remember, ejaculation is basically a two-step process. As arousal increases, you eventually reach the point of no return: ejaculatory inevitability. That is the moment when you feel that you are going to climax and there is nothing you can do about it. Physiologically speaking, you are correct; there *is* nothing you can do about it. Once that point is reached, the *ejaculation reflex* is set in motion, the muscles of the perineum forcefully contract, and the seminal fluid is already on its way out. In seconds, the expulsion stage is triggered. To delay ejaculation, you must be aware enough to do something *before* the point of inevitability sneaks up on you.

The first step is to pay close attention to physical sensations as you approach ejaculation. Just as you learned when to start braking your car as you approach a stop sign, you can learn to recognize when you are getting too close to the point of inevitability. That is the time to make adjustments. Some men try to distract themselves by thinking of anything besides what is going on: baseball, work, or anything nonsexual. Unfortunately, this is rarely effective. Even if it does slow down the process, it also separates you from the intimate connection of making love and ultimately detracts from your full enjoyment of the moment. A more effective and far more enjoyable technique is to alter the way you are thrusting at that point: change the angle, speed, or depth of your thrusts, which will shift the sensations away from the head of your penis (the glans, which is the most sensitive part), thereby delaying ejaculation. Intercourse does not have to be limited to deep, rapid thrusts. You can make love slowly. You can move in a circular motion or enter only partway. The variations are limitless. The secret is to pay attention to the sensitivities of your own body and then make the appropriate adjustments to your sexual technique.

You can also stop thrusting entirely. Try suspending motion for a while and just lying together with your penis fully penetrated. It is a great way to reduce arousal and prolong intercourse. It can also be wonderfully romantic. When you feel you can resume thrusting without ejaculating immediately, resume your motion slowly.

Another variable is to withdraw entirely. This "start and stop" method is often used by sex therapists. When you feel yourself nearing inevitability, simply pull out and rest. If your relationship is a good one, your partner should understand the need for this and welcome the opportunity to do other erotic things. This is the time for using your hands, lips, tongue, and any other body part that gives you pleasure while at the same time giving your penis a break from direct stimulation. When you resume intercourse, it will be that much more intense and your total time of penetration will increase. Do not be afraid of losing your erection if you stop thrusting or pull out entirely. You *might* lose it, but so what? It will come back with the right stimulation.

Squeeze Me, Please Me

One of the best methods of delaying ejaculation is the squeeze technique. When you feel you are close to ejaculation, withdraw your penis. Then grip the head of your penis (the glans) at the juncture where it meets the shaft, holding your thumb on the upper surface and your first and second fingers underneath. On the head, squeeze forcefully. This will delay the urge to ejaculate. The amount of pressure needed varies among men, but do not be afraid to squeeze hard. Your erect penis can withstand a great deal of pressure without injury. When the urge is gone, wait a moment or two before resuming intercourse. It is possible to partially lose your erection after the squeeze, but that is *usually* not a problem. If it happens, do not panic. Remain relaxed and confident, and your full erection will return shortly, especially if your penis has fresh stimulation.

The squeeze technique is time-tested. You can use it anytime you feel you are about to ejaculate. Just withdraw, squeeze, and then resume intercourse. The squeeze technique is the solution I recommend most often to my patients.

Some of my patients say they prefer to have their partner do the squeezing, but I have found it more reliable for the man to do it himself, since he is more familiar with his own penis and knows when and exactly how firmly to squeeze. This technique is also used by my colleagues in sex therapy *without intercourse* as a method of systematically reconditioning men with long histories of premature ejaculation. In this process, the woman stimulates the man as if masturbating him but stops and squeezes when he signals that he is about to ejaculate. You are welcome to try this— there is nothing like on-the-job training.

The Valsalva Maneuver

A technique for delaying ejaculation that does not require withdrawal is the Valsalva maneuver, which involves holding your breath and bearing down with your abdominal muscles as if you were going to relieve stuffed bowels. You obviously squeeze your anal sphincter at the same time, so that you do not *actually* move your bowels. This creates a marked increase in intra-abdominal pressure and will delay the ejaculatory mechanism. As with the squeeze technique, timing is critical. If you do it too soon, it will not help. If you wait too long, you might reach the point of no return and all the breathing, holding, and squeezing in the world will be futile. Some men continue thrusting while doing the Valsalva maneuver, while others find it more comfortable to stop for a moment until they feel they can resume without exceeding the threshold of inevitability.

If you follow the techniques I have outlined above, you should increase your penis power and extend your staying power significantly. Please bear in mind that no matter how much you improve your self-control, there will always be moments when you will ejaculate sooner than you would like. Do not get down on yourself if that happens. Don't feel embarrassed or ashamed. There is no need to apologize. If you ejaculate before your partner is satisfied, try other means besides intercourse to bring your partner to an orgasm. If you leave your partner frustrated, make up for it the next time. When you feel yourself slip into that zone where you lose control, do not resist the inevitable—just relax and enjoy it.

Eliminate Negativity and Self-Doubt

Whether it is directed at your sexuality or any other aspect of your life, *self-doubt* can wilt your penis power like frost on a rose petal. Therefore, eliminating any and all self-doubt should be your number one priority in your quest for superpotency.

A man who aspires to superpotency should not let himself succumb to negativity in any form. Of course you are not perfect. Of course you make mistakes. Of course you have some weak spots and insecurities. We all do. Denying that you have flaws is not a healthy response to challenges in your life. A superpotent man always faces his imperfections with honesty and humor. You should never let anything obscure the basic and unconditional acceptance of yourself.

If you see the proverbial glass as half full rather than half empty, your penis will *behave* accordingly. If you succumb to cynicism, pessimism, and despair, you will become an empty shell of negativity and hopelessness, and so will your penis. Every situation, sexual or otherwise, can be viewed through many lenses. It is up to you to respond to the realities of your life in a strong and confident manner, which then positively reinforces your self-esteem.

Act like a winner in life, and you will be a winner in bed. Face the world with courage, and your penis will be courageous as well. Go through life with a smile on your face, and your penis will smile as well. Extract every drop of pleasure that life offers you, and your penis will make you doubly happy.

It may take time and effort to cultivate the positive attitudes necessary for superpotency. For some men, old habits are hard to break, and negative thinking is just that, a habit. Your mind might be accustomed to focusing on the negative because you are afraid of letting your guard down. Some of us learned early on that if we expect too much from life, we end up disappointed or ambushed by fate. We may have learned to look at the negative as a kind of self-defense. Too often I have seen negativity become a self-fulfilling prophecy. The trick is to see reality for what it is, focus on your own positive traits, and have confidence in your ability to make the most out of any situation. If can you do this, your penis power will flourish.

Do Not View Sex as a Performance

As I have repeated throughout the book, *performance anxiety* is a sure way to produce penis weakness. If you stop thinking about sex as something you perform, as if it were a stage production, an athletic event, or an exercise on which you are being graded, you will eliminate performance anxiety. If you find yourself thinking about how you are going to do when you are in bed, you are on the wrong track. Alter that negative image immediately. Visualize yourself simply enjoying each and every moment of the anticipated sexual encounter. Do not clutter your mind with extraneous details. Go into it expecting nothing from yourself other than to experience pleasure and give pleasure. Simply put, just go with the flow. You should not be worrying about whether you are doing a good job or how you compare to other men. Remove all comparisons and all standards of performance from your mind. Take it as it comes, and pleasure will become a reliable outcome for both you and your partner.

Ultimately, the outcome does not matter. Your capacity to relax and enjoy the intimacy and romance of sex is all that matters. Your attitude toward your penis should be governed by the same positive reinforcement you would give to a child who is playing a soccer game or taking an exam: "I do not care if you win or lose. All that matters is that you give it your best shot."

Never let yourself be intimidated by a sexual partner. If she is too demanding, if her expectations are unrealistic, or if she compares you to other men, then that problem is *hers*, not yours. Never let an attitude of self-doubt inhibit you or make you doubt your performance. Yes, you have a responsibility to try your best to satisfy your partner, but all you can do is exactly that: give it your best effort. If you have done that, you have no reason to feel guilty or ashamed. Those negative emotions do not belong in the life of a superpotent man. The most important course of action you can take to develop a strong and prodigious sexual essence is to promote the qualities and habits that will make you the best man you can be.

Make Friends with Your Penis

Just as much as any other part of your body, your penis is out in the world representing you. It reflects what you think of yourself and your life. Love your penis. Respect it, treat it well, and take pride in it. Above all, have faith in it. Your penis is your friend. You should treat it accordingly.

If your penis has let you down at any point and you have come to mistrust it, then it is time to forgive it and move on. Take personal responsibility for previous failures. Do not attribute them to your penis. It is only an emissary that follows orders from your brain. Do not kill the messenger—just resolve the issues that may have caused the past problems. Your penis will behave the way you want it to if you treat it well and let it know you believe in it.

Nothing will invigorate you more than an enthusiastic attitude toward your penis. If self-doubt pops into your mind, defeat it with positive thoughts about yourself. Redirect your thinking to the things of which you are proud. Tell yourself, "My penis has my utmost confidence and support. It is my friend. It will serve me faithfully."

Spend some time alone with your penis. I do not necessarily mean masturbate. Take a good look at it in the mirror and see it for the beautiful, whimsical organ that it is. It is a court jester and a sage rolled into one. Its sole mission is to bring you happiness. Touch it, massage it with lotion, or sprinkle it with fragrance. There is no reason men should be ashamed to do such things. We treat our faces and the rest of our bodies with special care, so why not our genitals? Doing this will help you fortify the bond between your brain and your penis. Treat your penis with respect, and it will serve you with dignity.

A Final Word to Women

That last sentence can also be rephrased for women: treat his penis with respect and it will serve *you* with dignity. This chapter has been directed to men, but I sincerely hope that women will study it carefully and use the information to help the men in their lives achieve their superpotency. As stated earlier, women who know how to attend to their men's penises have better relationships and better sex. If you take some of the time you spend trying to look attractive to men and use it to directly satisfy their sexual needs (both mentally and physically), you will attain far greater fulfillment.

Knowing how easily such statements can be misconstrued and how sensitive matters between the sexes are today, I must stress that being a penis-oriented woman does not make you less than an equal to the men in your life. In fact, it elevates your status because you now have a greater degree of control and power in the relationship. Taking the time to understand what makes your man tick and learning to satisfy his penis needs does not make you subservient in any way. It simply means holding up your end of the relationship so that *your* needs are satisfied in return. By taking the initiative, you can establish a precedent that your man can be expected to follow *quid pro quo*.

More than thirty years of clinical experience have convinced me of this: an intelligent woman knows that one of the best ways to a man's heart and soul is through his penis.

A Final Word to Men

Penis power is not about size or the number of sexual conquests you have had. It is not about blood vessels and nerves. Rather, it is about heightened self-awareness. If you adopt an enlightened attitude that is enthusiastic, conciliatory, and understandingly assertive, your sexuality will follow. Penis power is about admiring and respecting a body part that is never out of style, can never be overused, and can never be worn out. It is about letting your penis read your mind and allowing your mind's voice to cry out, "My penis is *great*, and if it is great, *I am great*! It is Mr. Happy, and I am Mr. Happy!"

Penis power is a priceless luxury that is readily available to every man to be shared in every relationship throughout a lifetime of intimacy and compassion. Penis power is not about domination, but rather communication and sensitivity between lovers. It is about sharing the mystique of man's most enigmatic body part with understanding and enthusiasm. Penis power is about an emotional and sexual generosity that is *not* out of a need to achieve saintliness. The truth is that all intimate relationships should be dictated by mutually respectful self-interest—the more you give, the more you will receive in return. In reality, what most people really want from their lives is some form of happiness. If you can learn how to achieve mutual happiness with your partner, you will find that life truly is a beautiful experience.

Penis power is about reducing anxiety and enhancing the quality of your existence in every respect. It is about maintaining good health, exercise, diet, and attitude. It is about appreciating the penis you have, instead of having a penis you do not appreciate. It is realizing that your penis is one of life's greatest gifts and that penis power is your own personal achievement. This power is to be shared wisely with your mate, so that together you can soar to new heights of pleasure and intimacy.

As a penis doctor, I recommend that you stay as young as your penis. Use this book to develop communication skills with your penis. Whatever you do, *do not lose faith in your ability to improve your sexuality*. Love as well as you can because to love well is to live well. Share the pleasures of your penis as honestly and openly as you can, and you and your partner will be better off for it. Life is about more than eating and drinking and getting and spending. It is about cultivating a healthy mind and a healthy body and sharing that with the world. That is the essence of superpotency.

I truly believe that a wise man would rather be a pauper and use his penis like a king than be a king who is incapable of exercising and sharing his right to penis power.

Acknowledgments

Special thanks to my dear wife, Hedva, without whom none of this would be possible. I am grateful to my daughter, Aurele Danoff, for her invaluable perspective and support. Thanks to my son, Doran A. Danoff, for his editorial assistance and insights in helping to create this book. And an extra-special thanks to my longtime friend and professional colleague Dr. Leo Gordon for his impeccable sense of literacy and for his professorial advice in helping to edit the final draft of this book.

And dare I forget to thank the women who have influenced my life—both through my practice and personal endeavors—for their unique perspective and wisdom. They have allowed me to express my ideas with a passion not otherwise possible.

Notes

Chapter 1

1. *Macbeth: A Tragedy*, ed. Samuel Johnson and George Steevens (London: Mathews and Leigh, 1807), act 2, sc. 3.

Chapter 3

1. Staff of the Institute for Sex Research, Indiana University, *Sexual Behavior in the Human Female* (Bloomington, IN: Indiana University Press, 1953), 594.

Chapter 5

1. Surveillance, Epidemiology, and End Results Program, "SEER Stat Fact Sheets: Prostate," National Institutes of Health, http://seer.cancer.gov /statfacts/html/prost.html (accessed February 4, 2011).

Chapter 6

1. National Kidney and Urologic Diseases Information Clearinghouse, "Erectile Dysfunction," National Institutes of Health, http://kidney .niddk.nih.gov/kudiseases/pubs/impotence/ (accessed February 4,2011).

2. Hunter Wessells, et. al., "Erectile Dysfunction and Peyronie's Disease" in *Urologic Diseases in America* (Washington, DC: Government Printing Office, 2007), chap. 15. http://kidney.niddk.nih.gov/statistics/uda /Erectile_Dysfunction_and_Peyronies_Disease-Chapter15.pdf.

3. Chris Steidle, "Viagra, Levitra, Cialis for ED," Seekwellness.com, http:// www.seekwellness.com/mensexuality/viagra_update.htm (accessed February 4, 2011).

4. Ibid.

Chapter 7

1. Warren G. Bennis, *An Invented Life* (New York: Basic Books, 1994), 57.

2. Bertrand Russell, *The Conquest of Happiness* (New York: W. W. Norton & Company, 1996), 62.

Chapter 8
1. Menstuff.org, "Do You Ever Fantasize about Someone Else During Sex?," http://www.menstuff.org/columns/numbers/archive.html (accessed February 4, 2011).

Chapter 9
1. *Henry IV: Part II*, ed. Henry Hudson (Boston: Ginn & Company, 1888), act 2, sc 3.

Chapter 10
1. County of Los Angeles, "Annual Sexually Transmitted Disease Morbidity Report, 2000-2001," Department of Health Services, http://www.lapublichealth.org/wwwfiles/ph/dcp/std/stdmorb2001.pdf (accessed February 4, 2011).
2. National Institute of Allergy and Infectious Diseases, "Chlamydia," National Institutes of Health, http://www.niaid.nih.gov/topics/chlamydia/pages/default.aspx (accessed February 4, 2011).
3. National Surveillance Data for Chlamydia, Gonorrhea, and Syphilis, "Trends in Reportable Sexually Transmitted Diseases in the United States, 2004," Centers for Disease Control and Prevention, http://www.cdc.gov/std/stats04/trends2004.htm (accessed February 4, 2011).
4. Herpes Diagnosis, "How Do You Get Herpes Infections?" Herpesdiagnosis.com, http://www.herpesdiagnosis.com/infected.html (accessed February 14, 2011); New York Times, "Herpes Simplex," http://health.nytimes.com/health/guides/disease/herpes-simplex/overview.html (accessed February 14, 2011).
5. County of Los Angeles, "HIV/AIDS Surveillance Summary, January 2008," http://lapublichealth.org/wwwfiles/ph/hae/hiv/HIVAIDS%20semiannual%20surveillance%20summary_January2008.pdf (accessed February 14, 2011); Mark Cichocki, "AIDS / HIV Blog," About.com, http://aids.about.com/ (accessed February 5, 2011).

Chapter 12
1. Department of Health and Human Services, "Male Circumcision and Risk for HIV Transmission and Other Health Conditions: Implications for the United States," Centers for Disease Control and Prevention, http://www.cdc.gov/hiv/resources/factsheets/circumcision.htm (accessed February 4, 2011).

2. Centre for Genetics Education, "Fact Sheet 51: What is meant by a family history of prostate cancer?," http://www.genetics.com.au/factsheet/fs51.asp#para_4 (accessed February 4, 2011).

3. Richard Gallagher and Neil Fleshner, "Prostate Cancer: Individual Risk Factors," *Canadian Medical Association Journal* 159 (1998) 807–13, http://www.cmaj.ca/cgi/reprint/159/7/807.pdf.

4. Scott Kincade, "Testicular Cancer," *American Family Physician*, http://www.aafp.org/afp/990501ap/2539.html (accessed February 4, 2011).

Index

A

abnormal conditions, 10, 212, 218
addiction to sex, 217. *See also* substance
    use/abuse
adolescents
    arousal triggers in, 45
    information sources for, 8–9
    penis size and insecurity, 35
    premature ejaculation, 298–299
    problems in, 173–174
    teaching sons about penis power,
        209, 228–230
age factors
    attitude toward aging, 183–185
    awareness of, 170
    desire versus performance, 169
    force of ejaculation, 50
    incidence of prostate cancer, 90
    intensity of orgasm, 223–224
    longevity of penis power, 186–187
    peak period of sexuality, 174–175
    problems in adolescence/early
        adulthood, 173–174
    quality of life improvements, 188
    retarded ejaculation, 297
    testosterone levels, 178–179
    use of erectile dysfunction
        medications/devices, 187
    widowers and dating, 186–187
aggression, perceived, 103
alcohol use/abuse, 15, 73–74, 208, 291
alpha-blockers, 86–87
alprostadil (prostaglandin-E), 107–109
American Urological Association, 76
amphetamines, 75
anabolic steroids, 67–68
anal intercourse, 153–154
anatomy
    learning about, 275
    penis, 41–42, 214
    prostate gland, 84
    related to ejaculation, 49–50
    sperm production, 47–48
    testicles, 234

Androgel, 182
andropause, 67, 178–179, 181, 185–186
anger/hostility, 165–167, 250, 258
anti-androgens, 87
anxiety, 14–15, 17–18, 78, 283. *See also*
    performance anxiety
aphrodisiacs, 44, 74, 119–121, 166
appearance of penis, 26–28, 37–39,
    211–213
arm strength, 294–295
Armstrong, Lance, 95–96
arousal, 42–43. *See also* erotic stimulation
arterial insufficiency, 64
atmosphere/environment, 157–158
atrophy of testicles, 67–68
attitude(s)
    aging and, 176–177, 183–185
    importance/effects of, 126–127
    of leader, 271
    oral sex, 155
    penis, 230
    positive, 128
    readjusting, 285
    toward sexual behavior, 273–284
attractiveness, 266–269, 279–280

B

Barnard, Christiaan, 120
behavior
    attitudes toward sexual, 273–284
    goal-oriented, 204
    lying/deceptive, 281
    of partners, 132
    of penises, 6, 237–239 (*see also* Penis
        Personalities)
    relationship to self of penis's, 275
    risk-taking, 278
    of superpotent men (*see*
        superpotency)
benign prostate hypertrophy (BPH),
    83–85
Bennis, Warren, 127
birth control for men, 218–220. *See also*
    condoms
bladder, 84, 85

blood flow/volume
  blood vessels, 42
  cock rings and, 220
  diagnostic tests for, 64
  effects on penis power, 170
  erection problems caused by, 113–114
  during tumescence, 45
  vascular disorders, 63–64
  See also cardiovascular disease
blow jobs, 43, 118–119, 154–156, 159
blue pills. See erectile dysfunction medications
body image, 19, 27–28, 291–292
body language, 280–281
boredom with sex, 146, 148, 150–152
boundaries, establishing sexual, 205–206
BPH (benign prostate hypertrophy), 83–85
bulbocavernosus reflex test, 62–63

C
cancer
  genitourinary tract, 95
  penile, 226
  prostate, 83, 84, 90–95, 181, 226–228, 232–233
  survival rates, 92
  testicular, 95–96, 233
  urinary bladder, 233
cardiovascular disease, 63, 105, 180–181, 215–216
cardiovascular fitness, 291
casual sex, 18
catecholamine, 74–75
Caverject, 104
Centers for Disease Control (CDC), 189, 194, 257
cervical cancer, 193
character of superpotent men, 268–269
chest pain, 216
childbirth, 220–221
chlamydia, 190
chordee, 26
Cialis, 8, 37, 100
circumcision, 225–226
"clap," the (gonorrhea), 191
clumsiness during sex, 204–205
cocaine use, 74–75
cock rings, 220
coming. See ejaculation; orgasms
commonalities among men, 4

communication topics
  aging issues of sexuality, 185–186
  for avoiding assumptions, 178
  conflicts with partner, 166–167
  desire levels, 222
  diplomatic, 208–209
  doctor's discussions with patients, 8–10
  erectile dysfunction medications, 103
  establishing boundaries, 205–206
  hygiene issues, 160
  listening to your partner, 281
  Negative and Positive Penis Personalities, 263
  nonverbal, 207
  pain during sex, 204–205
  partner's sexuality, 289–290
  performance anxiety, 131–132
  physical needs, 212
  premature ejaculation, 77, 299–300
  teaching sons about penis power, 209, 228–230
  tips for women, 199–201
  with unresponsive partners, 161
  working out ground rules, 202
comorbidities. See risk factors and comorbidities
complaints, men's and women's, 11, 201–210
condoms, 79, 153–154, 195–196, 219
continence/incontinence, 92
control of your life, 284–285
Coolidge Effect, 146, 148–149
coronary artery disease, 180
corpora cavernosa, 38, 42
corpus spongiosum, 42
courage, 271
Cowper's glands, 48
crisis management, 293–294
"crutch effect," 125, 128
cystoscopy, 85

D
Danoff's Law, 208
dapoxetine (Priligy), 80
daVinci technology, 91, 227
deceptive practices, 281
depression, 80, 283
desire (libido), 66
  differences in partners', 201–202
  diminished, 55, 166
  drugs that diminish, 75

desire (*continued*)
  loss of, 185–186, 220–221
  normal/abnormal, 218
  versus performance, 169
  reasons for decline in, 96
  use of erectile dysfunction
    medications without, 101
detumescence, 46
diabetes, 65–66
diagnostic methods/tests
  bladder scan, 84
  bulbocavernosus reflex test, 62–63
  cystoscopy, 85
  Doppler pulse-wave analysis, 64
  nocturnal penile tumescence (NPT)
    test, 60–62
  penile arteriography, 64
  postage stamp test, 61
  for prostate cancer, 92, 232
  prostatic specific antigen (PSA), 90
  symptoms requiring, 231–232
diet/nutrition, 291–292
digital rectal examination (DRE), 84
Doppler pulse-wave analysis, 64
dose-optimized thermal therapy (DOT),
  87–88
DOT (dose-optimized thermal therapy),
  87–88
DRE (digital rectal examination), 84
drug abuse. *See* substance use/abuse
drugs/medications, 15
  for benign prostate hypertrophy, 86
  as cause of erectile dysfunction, 66,
    70–73
  for erectile dysfunction (*see* erectile
    dysfunction medications)
  interactions of, 106, 107
  male sexual enhancement, 8
  off-label use of, 80–81
  for premature ejaculation, 76, 79–80
  problems of self-medication, 72
  resistance to antibiotics, 190, 191
  side effects of, 70–72
  steroids, 67–68
dysfunction. *See* erectile dysfunction;
    impotence; medical conditions
    affecting sexual dysfunction

E
ego, 200
ejaculation, 17
  changes with age, 176

ejaculation (*continued*)
  controlling timing of, 296–300, 304
  delayed, 177–178
  detumescence after, 46
  drugs for controlling, 80
  frequency of, 173
  health benefits of, 233
  medications causing dysfunctional,
    70–72
  methods for delaying, 220
  orgasms versus, 46–47
  physiology of, 48, 49–50
  premature (*see* premature ejaculation
    [PE])
  refractory period following, 51–53
  spontaneous night, 297
  without orgasm, 47
  See also orgasms
ejaculation reflex, 10, 46–47, 49, 173,
  224, 298, 301
ejaculatory inevitability, 78
emotions
  anger/hostility, 165–167, 250, 258
  anxiety (in general), 14–15, 17–18,
    78 (*see also* performance anxiety)
  communicating, 281
  effects of negative, 283
  embarrassment/humiliation, 6–7, 16,
    18, 57, 128, 299
  guilt, 140–142, 150
  reflection in your penis of, 238
  understanding your, 271–272
  See also Penis Personalities;
    psychological issues
endocrine disease, 105
enhancement/enlargement of penis,
    myths about, 31, 37–39, 213
environment/atmosphere, 157–158
epididymitis, 190
erectile dysfunction
  age and, 76, 186
  aphrodisiacs, 119–121
  devices for, 100
  drugs for (*see* erectile dysfunction
    medications)
  hormonal causes, 65–67
  incidence of, 104
  injectable drugs for, 64–65
  with kidney failure, 96
  mechanical devices, 118–119
  medications causing, 70–73
  partial erections, 65

erectile dysfunction (*continued*)
  pelvic trauma and, 113
  prosthesis implantation, 38–39,
      114–118
  See also impotence
erectile dysfunction medications, 64–65
  with cardiovascular disease, 216
  cautions for using, 101–104, 120–121
  Cialis, 8, 37, 100
  combined with drug abuse, 107
  crutch effect of using, 125, 128
  diagnosis for choosing, 105
  emergency use, 125
  for erections regardless of
      stimulation, 104
  finding effective, 105–106
  herbal remedies, 119–120
  history of, 99
  hype about, 106–107
  injectable, 104, 109–113
  Levitra, 8, 37, 100
  long-term effects of, 106
  mechanisms of action of, 100–101
  Muse system, 107–109
  overuse of, 111
  patient response to, 112–113
  side effects, 112
  use by gay/bisexual men, 107
  Viagra, 8, 15, 100, 104
  See also drugs/medications
erections (tumescence)
  age and (*see* age factors)
  anatomy of, 42
  beyond four hours (priapism), 106–
      107, 111, 220
  catecholamine reuptake and, 74–75
  changes with age, 175
  firmness of, 73–74, 170
  loss of, 21, 126
  origins of stimulation for, 42–43
  pharmacological, 109 (*see also* erectile
      dysfunction medications)
  physiology of, 33, 45–46
  reducing, 111
  during sleep, 59–60
  variations in hardness/size of, 30–31,
      32–33
erotic stimulation
  combining types of, 34
  pharmacologic erections and, 110
  premature ejaculation and, 76
  during refractory period, 52

erotic stimulation (*continued*)
  through the senses, 43
  videos, 282
estrogen, 185–186
exercise(s), 216, 294–296, 300–304
experience. *See* sexual experiences
experimenting with sex, 148–149

F
failure of penis. *See* erectile dysfunction;
      impotence
fantasies, during sex, 147
fatigue, 151–152, 215
fears
  of disease, 142–143
  effects of, 135–136
  irrational, 142–143, 251
feedback loops, 282–283
fertility, 68
first-time sex, 149–150
flaccid penis, size variations, 31
flavors/taste, 44
foreplay, 11, 79, 149, 155, 178, 221,
      288–289
fractured penis, 214
functions of penis, 41
fun/work balance, 293

G
gay men, use of erectile dysfunction
      medications by, 107
genital herpes, 192–193
genitals
  hygiene, 159–160, 212, 226
  misinformation about, 7–10
  natural curiosity about, 25–26
genitourinary tract, cancers of, 95
glans (head of penis), 34, 41, 214–215,
      302–303
goal-oriented behavior, 204
goals, focusing on positive, 127–128
Golden Rule, 198
gonorrhea (the "clap"), 191
guilt, 140–142, 150

H
habits, 136, 137
happiness, 271–272
"hard dick syndrome," 147–150, 186,
      278
"hard on demand" myth, 152–153
head of penis (glans), 41, 303
health issues

health issues (*continued*)
  benefits of sex for, 21–22
  diet/nutrition, 291–292
  maintaining good, 290–293
  physical fitness, 177, 184, 290
heart disease. *See* cardiovascular disease
herbal remedies for erectile dysfunction, 119–120
herpes, genital, 192–193
high blood pressure (hypertension), 70–71, 72
HIV/AIDS
  causes/symptoms/transmission/treatment, 193–196
  circumcision and reducing, 226
  condom use with, 153–154
  fear of, 142–143
  prevention awareness, 22
  with syphilis, 191–192
  use of erectile dysfunction medications with, 107
  See also sexually transmitted diseases (STDs)
hormonal causes of erectile dysfunction, 65–67
HPV (human papilloma virus), 193
human form, interest in, 279–281
human papilloma virus (HPV), 193
humiliation/embarrassment, 6–7, 16, 18, 57, 128, 299
humor. *See* jokes/humor
hygiene
  communication about, 160
  men's genitals, 159–160, 212, 226
  women's genitals, 159–160
hypertension (high blood pressure), 70–71, 72
hypogonadism, 67, 179
hypospadias, 26

I
imagination, arousal and, 45
impotence
  alcohol and, 208–209
  chronic alcoholism, 74
  as indicator of systemic disease, 104–105
  medical causes, 56–62
  physiological versus medical causes, 56
  prostatectomy and, 85, 91
  temporary, 125, 145–146, 276–277

impotence (*continued*)
  See also erectile dysfunction
IMRT (intensity-modulated radiation therapy), 93
incompatible partners, 161–162, 290
incontinence/continence, 92
infection risks, 154. *See also* sexually transmitted diseases (STDs)
infertility, 190
informed consent, self-administered injections, 112
injuries to penis, 213–215
inner qualities of superpotent men, 268–269
insecurity, 6–7, 18–19
integration of self and penis, 274
intensity-modulated radiation therapy (IMRT), 93
intercourse
  problems of prolonged, 178
  size of penis/length of vagina, 34
  techniques for prolonging, 301–304
  women's pain during, 205
intimidation by partners, 162–165, 202–203, 306–307
irrational fears, 142–143, 251

J
jokes/humor, 5
  about lapses of penis power, 277
  appreciation of absurdities, 271–272
  bulls and cows story, 176
  foreplay, 221
  intimidation joke, 162
  penis size, 29
  playfulness during sex, 203–204
  as tension relievers, 132

K
Kegel exercise, 300–301
kidney transplants, 96
Kinsey, Alfred, 42

L
"leisure world syndrome," 186–187
Levitra, 8, 37, 100
libido. *See* desire (libido)
Lincoln, Abraham, 134
Los Angeles Department of Health Services, 194–195
lovers. *See* partners
lubrication, 48, 205
Lue, Thomas, 37

M

magnetic resonance imaging (MRI),
prostate cancer staging with, 92
male menopause. *See* andropause
marijuana use, 74
Martin, Lucien, 295–296
masculinity, 35, 212–214
Masters and Johnson method ("stop
start" technique), 80–81
masturbation, 17, 69, 79, 153, 172,
224–225, 297, 299
mechanical devices, for erectile
dysfunction, 118–119
medical conditions (in general)
diminishment of sexual activity due
to, 68–70
of sexual organs, 231–234
use of erectile dysfunction
medications with, 105, 110
use of mechanical erectile devices
with, 119
medical conditions affecting sexual
dysfunction, 23
diabetes, 65–66
diagnosing impotence for, 56–62
high blood pressure, 72
hormonal, 65–67
neurological, 62–63
prescription medications, 70–73
with retarded ejaculation, 297
vascular, 63–64
medications. *See* drugs/medications;
erectile dysfunction medications
menopause, 185–186. *See also*
andropause
mental health. *See* psychological issues
micropenis, 212
mind-set
importance of positive, 97
sex as performance, 306–307
superpotency, 274
morning erections, 60, 152–153
MRI (magnetic resonance imaging),
prostate cancer staging with, 92
mumps, 66–67
Muse system, 107–109
music, 157
mutual masturbation, 225
mystique of penis, 9
myths of male sexuality
"hard on demand" myth, 152–153
importance of penis size, 35

myths of male sexuality (*continued*)
penile enhancement/enlargement,
37–39, 213
penis size, 29
self-doubt and, 18–19

N

narcotics, 75, 107
National Institutes of Health (NIH),
104
Negative Penis Personalities, 249–263.
See also Penis Personalities
negative thinking, 136, 265–266
neo-synephrine, 111
neurological causes of impotence, 62–63
nicknames for penises, 5
nicotine, 75
nitric oxide, 101
nitroglycerine, 120
nocturnal emissions, 297
nocturnal erections, 59–60, 62–63
nocturnal penile tumescence (NPT) test,
60–62
nonsurgical treatment options, 87–90.
See also drugs/medications
normal conditions, 10, 19–20, 30–31
NPT (nocturnal penile tumescence) test,
60–62
nutrition/diet, 291–292

O

olfactory responses, 44, 158–160
oral sex/oral contact, 43, 118–119,
154–156, 159
orchitis, 66–67
organ-confined prostate cancer, 92–93
organic impotence, causes of, 56–62
orgasms
age-related changes, 177, 223–224
definition, 47
factors in satisfaction, 50–51
intensity of, 176
prolonging, 224
sensation of, 78
without ejaculation, 47
See also ejaculation

P

papaverine, 65
partial erections, causes of, 65
partners
anger/hostility toward, 165–167
annoyance with, 208

partners (*continued*)
  behavior of, 132
  caring for/about pleasure of, 281
  compatibility of size of penis and
    vagina, 34
  desire level discrepancies, 221–222
  disinterested/unresponsive, 160–162
  excitement of new, 148
  incompatible, 161–162, 290
  intimidation by, 162–165, 202–203,
    306–307
  relationship with, 139
  response to arousal of, 282
  as sex objects, 280
  swallowing/ingesting semen, 206
  understanding your, 288–289
  younger, 187
passion, reviving, 151–152
PDE-5 inhibitors, 79–81, 100–101, 106,
  107, 216
PE. *See* premature ejaculation (PE)
peak period of sexuality, 174–175
pelvic control exercise, 295–296
pelvic inflammatory disease, 190, 191
penile arteriography, 64
penile cancer, 226
penis
  appearance of, 26–28, 37–39,
    211–213
  aversion to partner touching, 207
  awareness/understanding of your,
    275
  behavior of your, 237–239
  being friends with your, 307
  changes with age to, 171–172 (*see also*
    age factors)
  hygiene for, 212
  micropenis, 212
  mystique of, 9
  odors of, 160
  personality of your (*see* Penis
    Personalities)
  size (*see* size of penis)
  social acceptance of, 28
  symbiotic relationship with, 274
penis envy, men's, 11
penis failure. *See* erectile dysfunction;
  impotence
"Penis Paradox," 135, 138, 149
Penis Personalities, 239
  Pampered Penis Personality, 258
  Paranoid Penis Personality, 257

Penis Personalities (*continued*)
  Passionate Penis Personality, 244
  Peaceful Penis Personality, 245
  Pedestrian Penis Personality, 255
  Peewee Penis Personality, 249
  Pensive Penis Personality, 243
  Perceptive Penis Personality, 240
  Percolating Penis Personality, 242
  Persistent Penis Personality, 241
  Perverted Penis Personality, 253
  Pessimistic Penis Personality, 249
  Petulant Penis Personality, 253
  Pharmaceutical Penis Personality,
    262
  Philanthropic Penis Personality, 243
  Phobic Penis Personality, 251
  Picky Penis Personality, 251
  Pile-Driver Penis Personality, 252
  Pioneer Penis Personality, 246
  Pious Penis Personality, 255
  Pipe-Dream Penis Personality, 254
  Pissed-Off Penis Personality, 258
  Plaintiff Penis Personality, 252
  Playful Penis Personality, 246
  Poetic Penis Personality, 247
  Political Penis Personality, 256
  Pompous Penis Personality, 254
  Pooped Penis Personality, 256
  Pornographic Penis Personality, 260
  Possessive Penis Personality, 259
  Powerful Penis Personality, 248
  Precocious Penis Personality, 247
  Preoccupied Penis Personality, 257
  Prepared Penis Personality, 242
  Principled Penis Personality, 241
  Procrastinating Penis Personality,
    260
  Prodigious Penis Personality, 248
  Professional Penis Personality, 261
  Profligate Penis Personality, 259
  Promiscuous Penis Personality, 250
  Protective Penis Personality, 244
  Psychedelic Penis Personality, 245
  Purposeful Penis Personality, 240
penis power
  after vasectomy, 218–219
  circumcision and, 226
  concept of, 23
  discovering your, 266–268
  exercises for, 294–295
  impact of physical conditions on, 97
  lapses of, 276–277

penis power (*continued*)
  self-awareness for, 308–310
  teaching sons about, 209, 228–230
  what defines, 284–285
  See also Positive Penis Personalities;
    superpotency
penis weakness
  boredom with routineness of sex and,
    147
  factors in epidemic of, 10–13
  reasons for, 14–21
  sudden onset of, 234
  See also erectile dysfunction;
    impotence; negative Penis
    Personalities; performance
    anxiety
penocentrism, 4–7
performance anxiety, 15
  absence of, 281–283
  age/experience and, 124–125
  communication with partner about,
    131–132
  effects of worry and fear, 135–136
  first time, 150
  focusing on positive versus failure,
    126–127
  guilt and, 140–142
  impotence due to, 123–124
  intimidation by partner and, 163–164
  as leading cause of penis failure, 126
  managing occasional, 128–131
  men's assumptions of deficiency,
    10–11
  overthinking sex, 306–307
  Penis Paradox and, 135, 138
  perseverance through, 133–135
performance
  age and (*see* age factors)
  frequency/quality of, 275–276
  viewing sex as, 306–307
  without prostate, 91
personality
  relationship to penis traits, 273
  self-perception of penis and, 7
  of your penis (*see* Penis Personalities)
phalloplasty, 37–39
pheromones, 44
physical attributes, 266–267
physical fitness, 177, 184, 290
physiology
  ejaculation, 48, 49–50
  erections, 33, 45–46

physiology (*continued*)
  learning about, 275
  of male sexual response, 77–79
  men's concerns about, 53
  refractory period, 51–53
  of scrotum, 51
  of sperm, 47–48
"pills, the." *See* erectile dysfunction
    medications
playfulness, 203–204
pleasure
  factors in, 50–51
  giving and receiving, 277–278
  sensation during orgasm, 49
  See also erotic stimulation
pornography, 19, 35, 225
positions
  for avoiding pain during intercourse,
    205
  finding creative, 206–207
  for oral sex, 155
  trying new, 153
  uncomfortable, 206
positive attitude, 127–128, 265–266
Positive Penis Personalities, 240–248.
    See also Penis Personalities
postage stamp test, 61
post-traumatic stress disorder (PTSD),
    293–294
potential, realizing your full, 269–270,
    284–285
premature ejaculation (PE), 21, 55, 75,
    297–298
  in adolescents, 173
  causes/frequency of, 75–76
  history of treatments, 80–81
  medications for, 80
  physiology of, 77–79
  psychosocial effects of, 76–77
  questions for self-determining, 78–79
  self-help techniques, 76, 79–80
  suggestions for, 297–300
  tain't exercise for, 300–301
  techniques for delaying, 301–304
prevention measures
  condoms, 79, 153–154, 195–196, 219
  HIV/AIDS, 22
  medical problems of sexual organs,
    231–234
  problems of prostate in general, 233
  prostate cancer, 94
priapism, 106–107, 111, 220

Priligy (dapoxetine), 80
prostaglandins, 65, 104, 107–109
prostatectomy, 85, 86–87, 91
prostate gland, 48
   benign prostate hypertrophy (BPH),
      83–85
   cancer of, 90–95, 181, 226–228,
      232–233
   enlargement of, 231–232
   maintaining health of, 291
   role of, 145
prostatic specific antigen (PSA) test,
      90, 232
prosthesis implantation, 38–39, 114–118
protease inhibitors, 107
psychological issues
   addiction to sex, 217
   aging (See age factors)
   causes of dysfunction, 58–59
   depression, 80, 139–140, 283
   effects of negative emotions, 283–
      284
   with erectile dysfunction, 103
   irrational fears, 142–143
   maintaining good mental health,
      293–294
   performance anxiety (see performance
      anxiety)
   psychotherapy for sexual dysfunction,
      13, 80–81
   treatment for premature/retarded
      ejaculation, 55–56
   visualization exercise, 136
   See also emotions; Penis Personalities
PTSD (post-traumatic stress disorder),
      293–294

Q

qualities of superpotent men, 266–267,
      268–273, 287
quality of life, 188
quality relationships, 272–273
"quickies," 207

R

radiation therapy, 93
recreational drugs. See substance use/
      abuse
refractory period, 51–53, 78, 146, 175–
      176, 223–224
rejection of sexual overtures, 202–203,
      280–281

relationships
   conflicts in, 165–167
   give and take in, 198, 308
   long-term, 150
   problems in, 16, 273
   quality, 272–273
   signs of problems in, 202–203
   symbiotic, with penis, 274
   with your partner, 139
   with your penis, 307
religious beliefs, 141–142
rest, 293
retarded ejaculation, 55–56, 297
rigidity (firmness of erection), 73–74,
      175
risk factors and comorbidities
   AIDS, 194
   anal sex, 153–154
   kidney failure, 96
   potential risks of testosterone
      replacement therapy, 179–182
   prostate cancer, 92, 181
risk-taking behavior, 278
romance, reviving, 151–152
routine sex, 147, 148–150, 152–153
Russell, Bertrand, 137

S

satisfaction
   expectation of, 15–16
   of female partners, 177
   having a satisfying sex life, 275–277
   size and, 34
scrotum, 51, 223
secret of penis power, 22–24
self-confidence/presence, 266, 269, 271
self-consciousness, 282–283
self-doubt, 13, 20, 128–129, 134, 225,
      230, 304–305
self-esteem
   chronic dysfunction and, 12–13
   perception of penis and, 6–7
   performance anxiety and, 124–125,
      128–130
   premature ejaculation and, 76–77
self-help techniques, for premature
      ejaculation, 80–81
self-image, 156, 239, 276, 292
semen (ejaculate)
   flavor/aroma of, 206
   production of, 47–48
   restoration after ejaculation of, 52

semen (ejaculate) (*continued*)
  swallowing/ingesting, 206
  volume of, 50, 51
seminal vesicles, 48, 52
sensate focus, 81
senses, effects on arousal by, 42–45
sensitivity of penis, diabetes and, 66
sepsis, 154
sex appeal, 266–267
sex drive, 11, 66
sex education, 17, 209, 228–230
sexual activity
  aging and (*see* age factors)
  attitudes and behaviors toward,
      273–284
  burning out your penis, 215
  businesslike, 203–204
  damage to penis through, 213–215
  diminishment due to illness, 68–70
  distasteful, 205–206
  heart disease and, 215–216
  initiation of, 202–203
  loss of interest in, 185–186
  men's demands/expectations for,
      201–202
  in new millennium, 188
  offensive/radical, 253
  overintellectualizing, 290
  as a performance, 306–307
  reasons for limiting/changing, 69–70
  for resolving grievances, 208
  routine, 147, 148–150, 152–153
  satisfying sex life, 275–277
  slowing down, 206–207
  unimaginative, 255
sexual dysfunction rates, 10–11, 12–13.
      See also erectile dysfunction;
      impotence; medical conditions
      affecting sexual dysfunction
sexual ennui, 150
sexual experiences
  elements of, 101
  enhancing with recreational drugs,
      73–75
  first times, 125
  psychological issues of, 103–104
  unsatisfactory, 218
  of your partners, 195
sexual inactivity, 298
sexuality
  being at ease with, 279–281
  in later years, 185

sexuality (*continued*)
  men's ignorance about, 288
  resignation to loss of, 171
  self-perception of penis and, 7
  understanding your partner's specific,
      289
sexually transmitted diseases (STDs),
      142–143
  chlamydia, 190
  genital herpes, 192–193
  gonorrhea, 191
  HIV/AIDS (*see* HIV/AIDS)
  incidence of, 189
  risk-taking behavior, 278
  syphilis, 191–192
sexual response cycle, 78
sinusoids, 42
size of penis
  adolescents' insecurity about, 35
  changes with age, 174–175
  enlarging procedures, 213
  of flaccid penis, 31
  men's weight and, 36
  myths about changing/improving,
      37–39, 213
  pain for women, 205
  physiological importance of, 33
  preoccupation with, 28–29
  relationship of superpotency to, 31–32
  variations in normal, 30–31
  women's concerns about, 211–213
smells, 44, 158–160
social conditions, as factors in penis
      weakness epidemic, 14
sounds, arousal with, 44
Spanish fly, 119–120
sperm, 47–48, 219
spicing up sex
  cautions for, 153–154
  different times and places, 156–158
  morning sex, 152–153
  mutual masturbation, 225
  oral sex, 154–156
  spontaneity and romance, 150–152
"squeeze" technique, 81
stage of life issues. *See* age factors
STDs. *See* sexually transmitted diseases
      (STDs)
steroids, 67–68
stimulation. *See* erotic stimulation
"stop start" technique (Masters and
      Johnson method), 80–81

stress
    compartmentalizing, 136, 138, 174
    knowing how to handle, 283–284
    management of, 137–138, 203
    medical consequences of, 14–15
    sex for alleviating, 138
subconscious, effects of, 157
substance use/abuse
    alcohol, 15, 73–74, 208, 291
    cocaine, 74–75
    ecstasy, 75
    with erectile dysfunction
        medications, 107
    marijuana use, 74
    narcotics, 75, 107
    Pharmaceutical Penis Personality,
        262
superpotency, 263
    as attitude of abundance, 266–268
    attitudes and behaviors toward sex,
        273–284
    character/quality of superpotent men,
        268–273
    definition, 23
    educating yourself for, 288–290
    eliminating self-doubt for, 304–305
    essence of, 309–310
    increases during summer, 222–223
    masturbation and, 224–225
    penis size and, 31–34
    teaching sons about, 209, 228–230
    working at, 134–135
    See also penis power
surgical procedures
    for erectile dysfunction, 113–114
    kidney transplants, 96
    for penis enhacement/enlargement,
        31, 37–39
    phalloplasty, 213
    prostatectomy, 85, 86–87, 91,
        226–228
    prosthesis implantation, 38–39,
        114–118
    for testicular cancer, 95–96
    total nerve-sparing prostatectomy,
        91, 93
Sutton's Law, 208
symbiotic relationship with penis, 274
symptoms needing urologic
        consultations, 231–232
syphilis, 191–192

T
tain't exercises, 300–301
"talk, the," 8
taste/flavors, 44
techniques for delaying ejaculation
    Masters and Johnson method, 80–81
    squeezing the glans, 81, 303
    stopping thrusting, 301–302
    Valsalva maneuver, 304
    withdrawing/pulling out, 302–303
temperature effects on superpotency,
        222–223
testicles
    atrophy of, 66–68, 217–218
    failure of, 67
    familiarity with structure of, 234
    production of sperm, 47
testicular atrophy, 66–68, 217–218
testicular cancer, 95–96, 233–234
Testim 1 percent, 182
testosterone, 66–67, 95–96, 178–179
testosterone replacement therapy
        (TRT), 178–182, 217–218
timing control, 296–300
touch, arousal with, 43
traits of your penis. See Penis
        Personalities
transdermal testosterone replacement
        therapy, 182
transplants, kidney, 96
transurethral microwave therapy
        (TUMT), 87–88
traumatic experiences, 293–294
treatment options
    after prostatectomy for cancer, 93
    alternatives to prostatectomy, 228
    for benign prostate hypertrophy,
        85–90
    diagnosing for successful, 61
    medical, 12
    for neurological conditions, 63
    of premature ejaculation, 79–81
    for prostate cancer, 90, 94
TRT (testosterone replacement therapy),
        178–182, 217–218
tumescence. See erections (tumescence)
TUMT (transurethral microwave
        therapy), 87–88
tunica, 42, 45–46

U
ultrasound, prostatic, 84

unpleasant aspects of sex, 159–162
unprotected sex, 153–154, 195–196.
    See also sexually transmitted
    diseases (STDs)
urethra, 42, 85
urethritis, 190
urination
    affects of benign prostate
        hypertrophy on, 83–86
    bladder, 84, 85
    continence/incontinence, 92
    medications for increasing, 71
    morning erections and, 60
    obstructions to flow, 83
urologic consultations, symptoms
    needing, 231–232

V
vacuum erectile devices (VEDs), 100,
    118–119
vagina, 159, 185–186
Valsalva maneuver, 304
vascular causes of impotence, 63–65
vas deferens, 48
vasectomies, 218–219
vasovasostomies, 219
VEDs (vacuum erectile devices), 100,
    118–119
venous leaks, 65, 113–114
"Venus envy," 224
Viagra, 8, 15, 100, 104
vibrators, as competition, 16
visualization exercise, 136
visual stimulation, 44

W
Wallenda Factor, 127–128
warts, genital, 193

weight control, 291–292
well-rounded lifestyle, 272
widowers, 186–187
winners, 270–271
women
    advice for, 197–198
    application of Penis Personalities to,
        263
    appreciation of penis by, 26–27
    avoiding infections, 154
    cervical cancer, 193
    childbirth effects on libido, 220–221
    chlamydia, 190
    communication about penises by, 26
    communication by, 199–201
    curiosity about penis, 11
    ectopic pregnancy, 190
    fantasies during sex, 147
    hygiene of, 159–160
    men's ignorance about, 288
    oral sex by and for, 154–156
    pain during sex, 204–205
    pelvic inflammatory disease, 190, 191
    penis-oriented, 209–210, 308
    penis preferences, 211–213
    priorities of, 32–33
    sexual and emotional suffering, 7
    sexually aggressive/intimidating,
        202–203
    sexual needs of, 15
    top ten complaints of, 201–210
    understanding of men's humiliation,
        57
women's movement, 15
work/fun balance, 293

Y
yohimbine, 120
youth cult, 292–293

About the Author

Dudley Seth Danoff, MD, FACS, is a diplomate of the American Board of Urology and a fellow of the American College of Surgeons. Born in Brooklyn, New York, Dr. Danoff is a graduate of Princeton University, summa cum laude and Phi Beta Kappa. He received his medical degree at Yale University with honors. He completed his urologic surgical training and fellowship at Columbia University Presbyterian Medical Center in New York City. Following his training, he served as a major in the United States Air Force Medical Corps. For more than a quarter century, Dr. Danoff taught on the clinical faculty of UCLA School of Medicine. Currently, he is attending urologic surgeon at Cedars-Sinai Medical Center in Los Angeles. He is the founder and president of the prestigious Cedars-Sinai Tower Urology Medical Group, the leading urologic practice serving the Southern California community for over thirty years. Dr. Danoff and his wife, Israeli singer Hedva Amrani, are longtime residents of Beverly Hills, California, and have two children: Aurele Danoff, an attorney, and Doran Danoff, a composer.